# The Complete Diverticulitis Diet Cookbook:

## 100+ Gut-Friendly Recipes & 8-Week Meal Plan for Digestive Wellness

D1518509

Alexandra Morgan

# TABLE OF CONTENTS

## Welcome to "Nourishing Choices: Your Diverticulosis-Friendly Cookbook"

This cookbook is designed with one primary goal: to help you enjoy delicious, satisfying meals while supporting your digestive health. Here, you'll find 115 recipes that cater to the dietary needs of diverticulosis and celebrate the joy of eating well.

### Understanding Diverticulosis

Diverticulosis occurs when small, bulging pouches (diverticula) form in the digestive tract, typically in the colon. While many people with diverticulosis experience no symptoms, others may face complications like diverticulitis – an inflammation of these pouches.

Diet plays a crucial role in managing diverticulosis. Generally, a high-fiber diet is recommended to promote regular bowel movements and reduce pressure in the colon. However, a temporary switch to low-fiber, easily digestible foods may be necessary during flare-ups. This cookbook caters to both scenarios, offering recipes for various stages of the condition.

### How to Use This Cookbook

Navigating the Recipe Sections

Our recipes are organized into six main categories:

1. Breakfast Bowls & Smoothies
2. Hearty Soups & Salads
3. Flavorful Main Courses
4. Deliciously Gut-Friendly Sides
5. Sweet Treats & Healthy Desserts
6. Snacks & Small Bites

Within each category, recipes are further divided based on the stage of diverticulosis:

- Week 1: Gentle Nourishment (for acute flare-ups)
- Week 2: Gradually Adding Back Fiber (for recovery phase)
- Maintenance: Balanced, fiber-rich recipes for everyday wellness

The cookbook also includes a comprehensive meal planning and prep section, featuring a 8-week meal plan with shopping lists, a batch cooking guide, and tips for eating out with diverticulosis.

### Adjusting Recipes

To make larger batches, multiply the ingredients by the desired servings. Cooking times may need slight adjustments.

### Navigating the Recipes

This cookbook is designed to support you through all stages of managing diverticulosis:

- For acute flare-ups: Start with recipes from Week 1 in Part 1 (p. 10-17)
- For the recovery phase: Progress to Week 2 recipes in Part 1 (p. 20-29)
- For ongoing maintenance: Explore the wide variety of recipes in Part 2 (p. 29-84)

For a structured approach to incorporating these recipes into your daily life, refer to our eight-week meal plan in Part 3 (p. 85-90).

### Building Your Diverticulosis-Friendly Kitchen

Essential Tools:

• High-powered blender or food processor
• Steamer basket
• Slow cooker
• Non-stick cookware
• Measuring cups and spoons
• Sharp knives

- Airtight containers

Key Pantry Staples:
- Whole grains (brown rice, quinoa, oats)
- Legumes (lentils, beans, chickpeas)
- Canned and frozen fruits and vegetables
- Lean proteins
- Herbs and spices
- Healthy cooking oils

## A Note on Nutritional Information

Throughout this cookbook, we provide estimated nutritional information for each recipe. However, please note that the amounts and brands of certain products may cause variations in the nutritional values shown. For the most precise information, we recommend using a nutrition calculator with the specific ingredients you've selected. This is particularly important when monitoring fiber intake or other nutritional aspects crucial to managing diverticulosis.

## A Note on Nutrition and Health

While this cookbook offers guidance, remember that everyone's needs are unique. Always speak with your healthcare professional before making big dietary changes for tailored counsel.

Now, let's embark on this culinary journey together. Here's to delicious meals and better digestive health!

# Frequently Asked Questions About Diverticulosis and Diet

**1. What exactly is diverticulosis?**

Diverticulosis is a condition where small, bulging pouches (diverticula) form in the lining of your digestive system, most commonly in the colon. It's quite common, especially as people age. Many people with diverticulosis don't have symptoms, but some may experience complications like diverticulitis.

**2. How does diet affect diverticulosis?**

Diet plays a crucial role in managing diverticulosis. A high-fiber diet is generally recommended to prevent complications, as it helps promote regular bowel movements and reduces pressure in the colon. However, during flare-ups, a temporary low-fiber diet may be necessary.

**3. Can I eat seeds and nuts if I have diverticulosis?**

Contrary to old beliefs, current research suggests that seeds and nuts do not increase the risk of diverticulitis flare-ups. They can be part of a healthy, high-fiber diet. However, if you notice that certain seeds or nuts trigger symptoms, it's best to avoid them.

**4. How much fiber should I aim for daily?**

The recommended daily fiber intake is 25 to 35 grams for most adults with diverticulosis. However, gradually increasing fiber intake is important to avoid digestive discomfort. Always seek individual guidance from your healthcare provider.

**5. Are there any foods I should always avoid?**

There's no universal list of foods to avoid for everyone with diverticulosis. However, during flare-ups, you may need to avoid high-fiber foods temporarily. Pay attention to your body and avoid any foods that consistently cause discomfort.

**6. How quickly can I transition from a low-fiber to a high-fiber diet?**

The transition should be gradual, typically over several weeks. Increase your intake of fiber-rich meals gradually, starting with tiny amounts. This allows your digestive system to adjust and helps prevent discomfort.

**7. Can probiotics help with diverticulosis?**

According to some research, probiotics may help maintain a healthy gut flora, which may benefit those with diverticular disease. However, more research is needed. Discuss with your doctor if probiotics might be right for you.

**8. How do I know if I'm having a flare-up (diverticulitis)?**

Severe stomach discomfort (typically on the lower left side), fever, nausea, and altered bowel habits are all possible signs of a flare-up. If you suspect a flare-up, contact your healthcare provider immediately.

**9. Is it safe to eat raw vegetables?**

Raw vegetables are safe and beneficial for most people with diverticulosis as part of a high-fiber diet. However, during acute flare-ups, your doctor may recommend avoiding raw vegetables temporarily.

**10. How often should I have check-ups for my diverticulosis?**

The frequency of check-ups can vary depending on your health situation. Generally, if you're not experiencing symptoms, routine colon cancer screenings may be sufficient. Discuss the appropriate check-up schedule with your healthcare provider.

While this cookbook offers broad nutritional recommendations, it's important to consult your physician or a certified dietitian for personalized guidance based on your specific health needs.

# Part 1: Weathering the Storm: Recipes for Acute Diverticulitis Flare-Ups

## Introduction to the Low-Fiber Phase

When you're experiencing an acute flare-up of diverticulitis, your digestive system needs a period of rest to heal. This is where the low-fiber phase comes in. It's a temporary dietary approach designed to reduce irritation and inflammation in your digestive tract.

## Why a Low-Fiber Diet?

During a flare-up, a low-fiber diet helps to:

1. Reduce bowel volume and movement, allowing inflamed areas to heal
2. Decrease the risk of blockages in inflamed diverticula
3. Minimize discomfort and pain associated with digestion

## What to Expect:

The low-fiber phase typically lasts a few days to a week, depending on your doctor's recommendations. You may start with clear liquids and gradually progress to low-fiber solid foods. It's crucial to follow your healthcare provider's guidance for this phase.

## Key Principles of the Low-Fiber Phase:

1. Choose easily digestible foods
2. Avoid raw fruits and vegetables
3. Opt for refined grains over whole grains
4. Limit dairy products
5. Avoid nuts, seeds, and tough meats
6. Stay hydrated with clear fluids

## Foods to Include:

- White bread, pasta, and rice
- Well-cooked, skinless, seedless vegetables
- Ripe bananas and melons
- Eggs
- Lean, ground meats
- Fish
- Smooth nut butters (in moderation)
- Low-fat dairy (if tolerated)

## Foods to Avoid:

- Whole grains
- Raw fruits and vegetables
- Nuts and seeds
- Legumes
- Tough meats
- High-fat foods
- Spicy foods

## Transitioning Out of the Low-Fiber Phase:

As your symptoms improve, you'll gradually reintroduce fiber into your diet. This transition should be slow and careful, adding one new food at a time to monitor how your body responds.

## Remember:

The low-fiber phase is temporary. While it's crucial for managing acute flare-ups, it's not a long-term solution. Once your symptoms have subsided, you'll work with your healthcare provider to transition back to a high-fiber diet, which is crucial for preventing future flare-ups and maintaining overall gut health.

The recipes in this section are designed to be gentle on your digestive system while still providing necessary nutrients during this sensitive time. Never alter your diet significantly without first speaking with your physician or a qualified dietitian, especially if you're experiencing a flare-up.

## 1. Soothing Bone Broth with Ginger and Turmeric

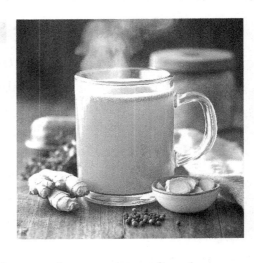

**Yields:** 2 servings | **Prep Time:** 10 minutes

**Cook Time:** 10 minutes (stovetop) or 6-8 hours (slow cooker)

**Ingredients:**

- 4 cups (960 ml) low-sodium chicken or vegetable broth
- 1-inch piece fresh ginger, peeled and thinly sliced
- 1 teaspoon ground turmeric
- 1/2 teaspoon sea salt, or to taste
- Freshly ground black pepper, to taste

**INSTRUCTIONS:**

**Stovetop Method:**

1. In a medium saucepan, combine the broth, ginger, turmeric, and salt. Bring to a simmer over medium heat.
2. Lower the heat to its gentlest setting, pop on the lid, and let the mixture simmer quietly for 10 minutes. This allows the ingredients to mingle and deepen their flavors. Once done, carefully pour the broth through a fine-mesh strainer into heat-safe vessels or serving bowls, catching any solid bits.

**Slow Cooker Method:**

1. Combine all ingredients in a slow cooker.
2. Cover the slow cooker with its lid and adjust the setting to the lowest temperature option. Let the ingredients simmer and cook for 6 to 8 hours, until the flavors have fully combined and developed.
3. Ladle the hot broth into mugs or bowls. Give your dish a personal twist by adding freshly cracked black pepper to suit your taste buds. Consult with your healthcare provider before adding black pepper or other spices to your diet. During these periods, it may be best to omit the black pepper from this recipe.

**Nutrition Per Serving:** Calories: 40 | Total Fat: 1g | Saturated Fat: 0g | Cholesterol: 5mg | Sodium: 480mg

Total Carbohydrate: 7g | Dietary Fiber: 0g | Sugars: 1g | Protein: 2g

## 2. Clear Chicken Broth with Soft Noodles

**Yields:** 2 servings | **Prep Time:** 5 minutes | **Cook Time:** 15 minutes

**Ingredients:**

- 4 cups (960 ml) low-sodium chicken broth
- 1/4 cup (25g) fine egg noodles or well-cooked white rice
- 1/2 cup (25g) shredded cooked chicken breast (optional)
- Salt to taste (if needed)

**INSTRUCTIONS:**

1. Heat a medium pot with the chicken stock until it simmers gently.
2. Add the egg noodles to the simmering broth. Reduce heat to low and cook until the noodles are very soft, about 8-10 minutes or according to package instructions.
3. If including chicken, gently stir in the shredded cooked chicken and heat through for 1-2 minutes.
4. Taste the broth and add a small amount of salt if necessary. Ladle into bowls and serve warm.

**Nutrition Per Serving (without chicken):** Calories: 70 | Total Fat: 1g | Saturated Fat: 0g | Cholesterol: 15mg | Sodium: 460mg | Total Carbohydrate: 10g | Dietary Fiber: 0g | Sugars: 1g | Protein: 5g

## 3. Egg Drop Soup

**Yields:** 2 servings | **Prep Time:** 5 minutes | **Cook Time:** 10 minutes

**Ingredients:**

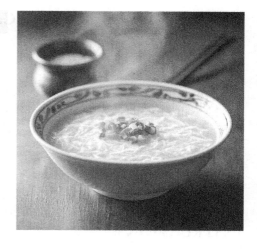

- 3 cups (720ml) low-sodium chicken broth
- 1/4 teaspoon (1.5g) salt
- 1/8 teaspoon (0.25g) white pepper
- 1/2 teaspoon (2.5ml) sesame oil
- 1 tablespoon (8g) cornstarch
- 2 tablespoons (30ml) cold water
- 2 large eggs, lightly beaten
- 1 green onion, thinly sliced (optional, for garnish)

**INSTRUCTIONS:**

1. Using a medium-sized pot, warm the chicken broth over medium heat until you see small bubbles forming around the edges. Once the broth is gently simmering, season it with a pinch of salt, a dash of white pepper, and a few drops of sesame oil for flavor.
2. Combine the cornstarch and cold water in a separate small container, stirring vigorously with a fork or whisk until you achieve a lump-free mixture.
3. Slowly stir the cornstarch slurry into the simmering broth. Stir until the soup slightly thickens, about 1-2 minutes.
4. Lower the heat to its minimum setting. Gradually drizzle the whisked eggs into the simmering broth, using a fork or chopsticks to gently stir the liquid in a circular motion as you pour. You'll notice the eggs cooking instantly, creating fine, ribbon-like strands throughout the soup.
5. Remove from heat. Taste and adjust seasoning if necessary. Distribute the soup into individual serving bowls and, if desired, sprinkle freshly chopped green onions on top for added flavor and visual appeal.

**Nutrition Per Serving:** Calories: 90 | Total Fat: 5g | Saturated Fat: 1.5g | Cholesterol: 185mg | Sodium: 420mg
Total Carbohydrate: 4g | Dietary Fiber: 0g | Sugars: 0g | Protein: 8g

## 4. Tofu and Broth Soup

**Yields:** 2 servings | **Prep Time:** 10 minutes | **Cook Time:** 15 minutes

**Ingredients:**

- 4 cups (960ml) low-sodium chicken or vegetable broth
- 1 package (14 ounces or 400g) soft tofu, drained and cut into 1-inch cubes
- 1 tablespoon soy sauce (low-sodium if available)
- 1/4 teaspoon ground ginger
- 2 green onions, white parts only, finely chopped (optional)
- Salt to taste, if needed

**INSTRUCTIONS:**

1. Heat a medium saucepan over medium heat and gently boil the broth.
2. Stir in the soy sauce and ground ginger. Taste and add a small amount of salt if needed, keeping in mind that the soy sauce already provides saltiness.
3. Carefully add the cubed tofu to the simmering broth. Reduce heat to low and let it cook gently for about 5 minutes, allowing the tofu to heat through without breaking apart.
4. In the final minute of cooking, add the chopped white sections of the green onions, if using. Remove from heat.
5. Ladle the soup into bowls, ensuring each serving has an equal distribution of tofu and broth.

**Nutrition Per Serving:** Calories: 180 | Total Fat: 9g | Saturated Fat: 1.5g | Cholesterol: 0mg | Sodium: 680mg
Total Carbohydrate: 5g | Dietary Fiber: 1g | Sugars: 1g | Protein: 18g

# 5. Pureed Carrot Soup

**Yields:** 2 servings | **Prep Time:** 10 minutes | **Cook Time:** 25 minutes

**Ingredients:**

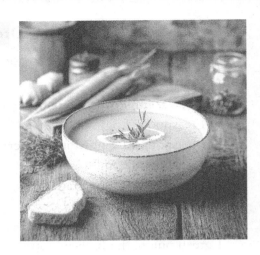

- 1 pound (450g) carrots, peeled and chopped
- 1 small onion, peeled and chopped
- 2 cups (480ml) low-sodium chicken or vegetable broth
- 1/2 cup (120ml) water
- 1 tablespoon olive oil
- 1/4 teaspoon salt, or to taste
- 1/8 teaspoon ground ginger (optional)

**INSTRUCTIONS:**

1. In a medium saucepan, warm the olive oil over medium heat. Cook the chopped onion for 3-4 minutes or until tender but not browned.
2. Add the chopped carrots to the pan and stir to combine with the onions. Pour in the broth and water. After bringing the mixture to a boil, turn down the heat. Cover and boil for about 20 minutes, until a fork easily pierces the carrots.
3. Remove the pan from heat. Using an immersion blender, carefully puree the soup until completely smooth. Alternatively, let the soup cool slightly and puree in batches in a standard blender.
4. Stir in the salt and ground ginger (if using). Taste and adjust seasoning if needed. If the soup is too thick, thin it with a little warm water or broth. Serve hot in bowls.

**Nutrition Per Serving:** Calories: 140 | Total Fat: 7g | Saturated Fat: 1g | Cholesterol: 0mg | Sodium: 400mg
Total Carbohydrate: 18g | Dietary Fiber: 5g | Sugars: 8g | Protein: 3g

# 6. Gelatin with Pear Juice

**Yields:** 2 servings | **Prep Time:** 5 minutes | **Chill Time:** 4 hours or overnight

**Ingredients:**

- 1 envelope (1/4 ounce or 7g) unflavored gelatin powder
- 1/4 cup (60ml) cold water
- 1 3/4 cups (420ml) pear juice, divided
- 1 tablespoon honey (optional)

**INSTRUCTIONS:**

1. In a small bowl, sprinkle the gelatin over 1/4 cup of cold water. Allow it to stand for 5 minutes so the gelatin can absorb the water and soften.
2. In a small saucepan, warm 3/4 cup of the pear juice over medium heat until it's hot but not boiling.
3. Remove the warm juice from heat and add the softened gelatin mixture. Stir until the gelatin is completely dissolved.
4. Pour the gelatin mixture into a medium bowl. Add the remaining 1 cup of pear juice and honey (if using). Stir until well combined.
5. Divide the mixture between two serving bowls or ramekins. Cover with plastic wrap and refrigerate for at least 4 hours or overnight, until the gelatin is fully set.
6. Once set, serve the gelatin chilled.

**Nutrition Per Serving:** Calories: 70 | Total Fat: 0g | Saturated Fat: 0g | Cholesterol: 0mg | Sodium: 10mg
Total Carbohydrate: 17g | Dietary Fiber: 0g | Sugars: 15g | Protein: 2g

## 7. Steamed Zucchini Puree

**Yields:** 2 servings | **Prep Time:** 10 minutes | **Cook Time:** 15 minutes

**Ingredients:**

- 2 medium zucchinis (about 1 pound or 450g), ends trimmed and chopped
- 1 tablespoon olive oil or unsalted butter
- 1/4 teaspoon salt, or to taste
- 1/8 teaspoon white pepper (optional)
- 2 tablespoons water or low-sodium chicken broth (if needed for consistency)

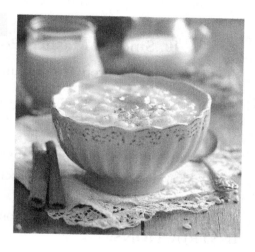

### INSTRUCTIONS:

1. Place the chopped zucchini in a steamer basket over a pot of simmering water. Cover and steam for 10-12 minutes, or until the zucchini is tender when pierced with a fork.
2. Once cooked, transfer the zucchini to a colander and let it drain for a few minutes to remove excess moisture.
3. Place the steamed zucchini in a food processor or blender. Add the olive oil or butter, salt, and white pepper (if using). Process until smooth, scraping down the sides as needed.
4. If the puree is too thick, add water or broth, one tablespoon at a time, until desired consistency is reached.
5. Transfer the puree to a serving bowl and serve warm.

**Nutrition Per Serving:** Calories: 80 | Total Fat: 7g | Saturated Fat: 1g | Cholesterol: 0mg | Sodium: 300mg Total Carbohydrate: 5g | Dietary Fiber: 1g | Sugars: 3g | Protein: 2g

## 8. Well-Cooked Rice Pudding

**Yields:** 2 servings | **Prep Time:** 5 minutes | **Cook Time:** 30-35 minutes

**Ingredients:**

- 1/2 cup (100g) short-grain white rice
- 2 cups (480ml) whole milk
- 2 tablespoons (25g) granulated sugar
- 1/4 teaspoon (0.5g) ground cinnamon
- 1/8 teaspoon (0.5g) salt
- 1/2 teaspoon (2.5ml) vanilla extract
- 1 tablespoon (14g) unsalted butter
- 2 tablespoons (30ml) heavy cream (optional)
- Ground cinnamon for garnish (optional)

### INSTRUCTIONS:

1. Rice, milk, sugar, cinnamon, and salt should all be combined in a medium saucepan.
2. Bring the mixture to a gentle simmer over medium heat, stirring frequently. Lower the temperature to its minimum setting and allow the mixture to cook without a lid for about 25 to 30 minutes. Remember to stir the pot regularly to ensure the rice doesn't adhere to the pan's base.
3. Your rice pudding is ready when the grains have become tender and the overall mixture has reached a thick, creamy consistency. If needed, cook for an additional 5 minutes.
4. After taking the pot off the heat source, incorporate the vanilla extract and butter into the pudding, mixing continuously until the butter has completely melted and blended into the mixture.
5. Let the pudding cool for about 5 minutes. As the pudding rests, you'll notice its consistency becoming even more substantial.

**Nutrition Per Serving:** Calories: 290 | Total Fat: 10g | Saturated Fat: 6g | Cholesterol: 30mg | Sodium: 200mg Total Carbohydrate: 43g | Dietary Fiber: 0g | Sugars: 18g | Protein: 7g

## 9. White Rice Congee with Chicken

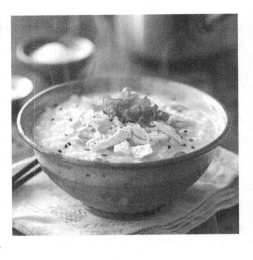

**Yields:** 2 servings | **Prep Time:** 10 minutes | **Cook Time:** 1 hour

**Ingredients:**

- 1/2 cup (90g) white rice, rinsed
- 4 cups (960 ml) low-sodium chicken broth
- 1 cup (240 ml) water
- 1 boneless, skinless chicken breast (about 6 ounces)
- 1/2 teaspoon salt, or to taste
- 1/4 teaspoon ground white pepper, or to taste

**INSTRUCTIONS:**

1. In a large pot or Dutch oven, combine the rinsed rice, chicken broth, water, chicken breast, salt, and white pepper.
2. Bring the mixture to a boil over medium-high heat.
3. Lower the heat to its gentlest setting, place a lid on the pot, and let it simmer quietly for 1 hour or until the rice has softened and partially dissolved, creating a thick, creamy congee texture to your preference. Stir occasionally to prevent sticking.
4. Remove the chicken breast from the pot and shred it using two forks.
5. Ladle the hot congee into bowls. Divide the shredded chicken among the bowls.

**Nutrition Per Serving (without toppings):** Calories: 250 | Total Fat: 3g | Saturated Fat: 1g | Cholesterol: 50mg Sodium: 600mg Total Carbohydrate: 35g | Dietary Fiber: 1g | Sugars: 0g | Protein: 25g

## 10. Smooth Mashed Potatoes (Without Skin)

**Yields:** 2 servings | **Prep Time:** 10 minutes | **Cook Time:** 15-20 minutes

**Ingredients:**

- 2 medium russet potatoes (about 1 pound/450g) peeled and cut into 1-inch cubes
- 1/4 cup (60ml) whole milk or unsweetened plant-based milk
- 2 tablespoons (30g) unsalted butter or olive oil
- 1/4 teaspoon salt, or to taste
- 1/8 teaspoon white pepper (optional)

**INSTRUCTIONS:**

1. Place the peeled and cubed potatoes in a medium saucepan and cover with cold water. Bring to a boil over high heat, then reduce to medium-low and simmer for 15-20 minutes or until the potatoes are tender when pierced with a fork.
2. Once cooked, drain the potatoes thoroughly in a colander. Return them to the hot pan and let them steam dry for about 1 minute, gently shaking the pan occasionally.
3. Add the milk, butter or olive oil, salt, and pepper (if using) to the potatoes. Using a potato masher or electric mixer, mash the potatoes until they reach a smooth, creamy consistency with no lumps.
4. Transfer the mashed potatoes to serving bowls and serve immediately while warm.

**Nutrition Per Serving:** Calories: 220 | Total Fat: 9g | Saturated Fat: 5g | Cholesterol: 25mg | Sodium: 320mg Total Carbohydrate: 32g | Dietary Fiber: 2g | Sugars: 2g | Protein: 4g

# 11. Well-Cooked White Rice

**Yields:** 2 servings | **Prep Time:** 5 minutes | **Cook Time:** 20-25 minutes

**Ingredients:**

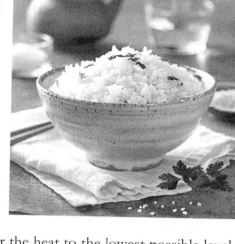

- 1 cup (190g) white long-grain rice
- 2 1/4 cups (540ml) water
- 1/4 teaspoon salt (optional)
- 1 teaspoon unsalted butter or olive oil (optional)

## INSTRUCTIONS:

1. Rinse the rice in a fine-mesh strainer with cold water for 30 seconds to 1 minute or until the water runs clear.
2. In a medium saucepan, combine the rinsed rice, water, and salt (if using).
3. Bring the mixture to a boil over high heat. After it comes to a boil, lower the heat to the lowest possible level, place a tight-fitting lid on the pan, and simmer it gently for 20 to 25 minutes. Avoid lifting the lid during cooking.
4. Once the cooking time has passed, remove the pan from the heat and let it stand, covered, for 5 minutes. In this way, whatever moisture that is left can be absorbed by the rice.
5. Gently fluff the rice with a fork, incorporating the butter or olive oil if using. Serve warm.

**Nutrition Per Serving:** Calories: 180 | Total Fat: 0g | Saturated Fat: 0g | Cholesterol: 0mg | Sodium: 150mg Total Carbohydrate: 40g | Dietary Fiber: 0g | Sugars: 0g | Protein: 3g

# 12. Soft-Boiled Eggs on White Toast

**Yields:** 2 servings | **Prep Time:** 5 minutes | **Cook Time:** 6-7 minutes

**Ingredients:**

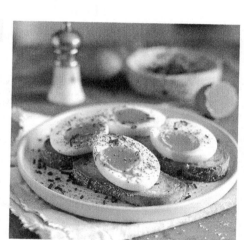

- 4 large eggs
- 2 slices of white bread
- 1 teaspoon unsalted butter or margarine (optional)
- Salt, to taste
- Freshly ground black pepper, to taste (optional)

## INSTRUCTIONS:

1. Fill a medium saucepan with enough water to cover the eggs by about an inch. Bring the water to a gentle boil over medium-high heat.
2. Gently lower the eggs into the boiling water using a slotted spoon. Reduce heat to maintain a gentle simmer and cook for 6-7 minutes for soft-boiled eggs.
3. While the eggs are cooking, toast the bread slices until lightly golden and crisp.
4. When the eggs are done, immediately transfer them to a bowl of cold water to stop the cooking process. Let them cool for about 1 minute.
5. Gently crack and peel the eggs. Place two eggs on each slice of toast. Before adding the eggs, if preferred, apply a thin coating of butter on the toast. Season with a pinch of salt and pepper if tolerated.

**Nutrition Per Serving:** Calories: 230 | Total Fat: 11g | Saturated Fat: 3g | Cholesterol: 370mg | Sodium: 280mg Total Carbohydrate: 20g | Dietary Fiber: 1g | Sugars: 2g | Protein: 15g

## 13. Simple Poached Salmon

**Yields:** 2 servings | **Prep Time:** 5 minutes | **Cook Time:** 8-10 minutes

**Ingredients:**

- 2 (4-ounce) skinless salmon fillets
- 2 cups (480ml) vegetable broth
- 1/4 teaspoon sea salt, or to taste
- 1 lemon, sliced (optional, for garnish)

**INSTRUCTIONS:**

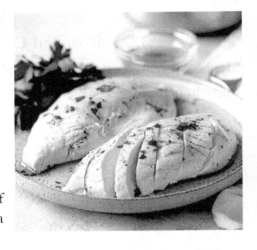

1. Gently pat the salmon fillets dry with paper towels.
2. Heat a large shallow pan over medium heat and gently boil the broth. Carefully slide the salmon fillets into the liquid. Reduce heat to low, cover the pan, and let the fish cook for 8-10 minutes or until it easily flakes with a fork.
3. Once cooked, remove the salmon from the broth using a slotted spoon. Season lightly with salt to taste.
4. Transfer the salmon to plates. Garnish with a slice of lemon if desired, but avoid eating the lemon during severe flare-ups.

**Nutrition Per Serving:** Calories: 233 | Total Fat: 14g | Saturated Fat: 3g | Cholesterol: 62mg | Sodium: 200mg
Total Carbohydrate: 0g | Dietary Fiber: 0g | Sugars: 0g | Protein: 25g

## 14. Plain Poached Chicken Breast

**Yields:** 2 servings | **Prep Time:** 5 minutes | **Cook Time:** 15-20 minutes

**Ingredients:**

- 2 (6-ounce) boneless, skinless chicken breasts
- 4 cups (960 ml) low-sodium chicken broth or water
- 1/2 teaspoon salt
- 2 sprigs fresh parsley (optional)

**INSTRUCTIONS:**

1. In a medium saucepan, combine the chicken broth or water with salt. If using, add the parsley sprigs. Transfer the liquid over medium heat to a moderate simmer.
2. Carefully lower the chicken breasts into the simmering liquid. Ensure they're fully submerged. Reduce the heat to low, cover the pan, and let the chicken cook gently for 15-20 minutes or until the internal temperature reaches 165°F (74°C).
3. Using a slotted spoon, remove the chicken from the cooking liquid and let it rest for 5 minutes. Slice or shred the chicken as desired and serve warm.

**Nutrition Per Serving:** Calories: 180 | Total Fat: 4g | Saturated Fat: 1g | Cholesterol: 85mg | Sodium: 420mg
Total Carbohydrate: 0g | Dietary Fiber: 0g | Sugars: 0g | Protein: 35g

## 15. Tender Flaked White Fish

**Yields:** 2 servings | **Prep Time:** 5 minutes | **Cook Time:** 10-12 minutes

**Ingredients:**

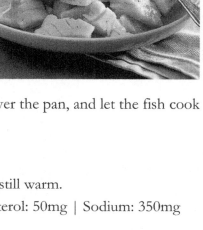

- 2 (4-ounce) fillets of white fish (such as cod, haddock, or tilapia)
- 2 cups (480ml) vegetable broth
- 1 bay leaf (optional)
- 1/4 teaspoon salt, or to taste
- 1 tablespoon fresh lemon juice (optional)

**INSTRUCTIONS:**

1. In a large, shallow pan, combine the broth, bay leaf (if using), and salt. Transfer the liquid over medium heat to a moderate simmer.
2. Carefully slide the fish fillets into the simmering liquid. Reduce heat to low, cover the pan, and let the fish cook for 8-10 minutes or until it easily flakes with a fork.
3. After the fish is done, move it to a platter with a slotted spoon.
4. Gently flake the fish with a fork. If using, drizzle with fresh lemon juice.
5. Divide the flaked fish between two serving plates and serve immediately while still warm.

**Nutrition Per Serving:** Calories: 100 | Total Fat: 1g | Saturated Fat: 0g | Cholesterol: 50mg | Sodium: 350mg

Total Carbohydrate: 0g | Dietary Fiber: 0g | Sugars: 0g | Protein: 22g

## 16. Steamed White Fish with Lemon

**Yields:** 2 servings | **Prep Time:** 5 minutes | **Cook Time:** 10-12 minutes

**Ingredients:**

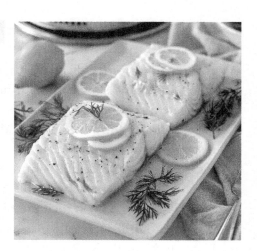

- 2 white fish fillets (about 6 ounces/170g each), such as cod, haddock, or tilapia
- 1 lemon, thinly sliced
- 2 teaspoons (10ml) olive oil
- 1/4 teaspoon (1.5g) salt
- 1/4 teaspoon (0.5g) black pepper
- 2 sprigs fresh dill (or 1 teaspoon/2g dried dill)
- 2 tablespoons (8g) fresh parsley, chopped (for garnish)

**INSTRUCTIONS:**

1. Set up a steamer basket over a pot of simmering water. Make sure the water doesn't touch the bottom of the basket.
2. Pat the fish fillets dry with paper towels. Drizzle a thin layer of olive oil over each fillet, then sprinkle with a pinch of salt and freshly ground pepper.
3. Place a few lemon slices in the steamer basket, then lay the fish fillets on top. Place the remaining lemon slices and dill sprigs on the fish.
4. Place a lid on the steamer and let the fish cook for about 10 to 12 minutes. Check for doneness by gently pressing a fork into the thickest part of the fillet; it should separate into flakes with little resistance. Remember that the cooking duration may vary depending on how thick your fish fillets are.
5. Carefully transfer the fish to plates, along with the lemon slices. Garnish with fresh parsley and serve immediately.

**Nutrition Per Serving:** Calories: 180 | Total Fat: 5g | Saturated Fat: 1g | Cholesterol: 65mg | Sodium: 360mg

Total Carbohydrate: 2g | Dietary Fiber: 1g | Sugars: 1g | Protein: 30g

# Week 2: Gradually Adding Back Fiber

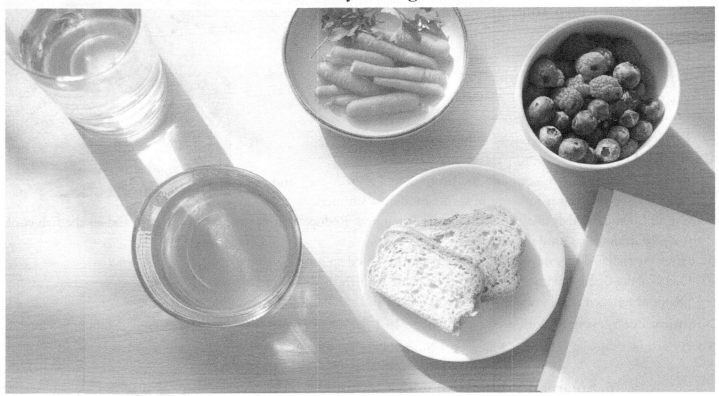

## Transition Guide: Moving from Week 1 To Week 2

As you recover from a diverticulitis flare-up, it's time to gradually reintroduce more fiber into your diet. This transition should be slow and mindful to avoid irritating your digestive system. Here are some guidelines to help you navigate this important phase:

1. Pace Yourself: Introduce new foods one at a time, in small amounts. This allows you to monitor how your body responds to each addition.

2. Increase Fiber Gradually: Aim to increase your daily fiber intake by 5-10 grams per week. The recipes in this section will help you achieve this goal safely.

3. Stay Hydrated: As you increase fiber, it's crucial to drink plenty of water. To aid in the digestion of the extra fiber, try to drink at least 8 glasses (64 ounces) of water daily.

4. Listen to Your Body: Pay attention to how you feel after eating. If you experience discomfort, return to Week 1 recipes for a day or two before trying again.

5. Chew Thoroughly: Take your time eating and chew your food well. This aids in digestion and helps your body adjust to the increased fiber content.

6. Cooking Methods: Continue to choose gentle cooking methods like steaming, boiling, and baking. You can progressively add a wider variety of cooking techniques as you advance.

7. Portion Control: Start with smaller portions of the new recipes and increase as tolerated.

8. Supplement Wisely: If recommended by your healthcare provider, consider taking a probiotic to support your digestive health during this transition.

9. Keep a Food Diary: Record what you eat and any symptoms you experience. This can help you identify which foods agree with you and which might need more time before reintroduction.

10. Consult Your Healthcare Provider: Always follow the specific advice of your doctor or dietitian. They may have personalized recommendations based on your individual health needs.

Everyone's digestive system is different, and what works for one person may not work for another. Be patient with your body as you navigate this transition. If you experience any persistent discomfort or concerning symptoms, contact your healthcare provider immediately.

## 17. Scrambled Eggs with Spinach (1g fiber per serving)

**Fiber Content:** 1g per serving | **Yields:** 2 servings | **Prep Time:** 5 minutes
**Cook Time:** 5 minutes

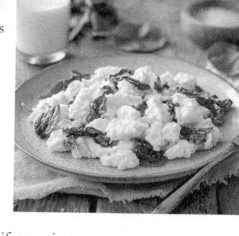

**Ingredients:**

- 4 large eggs
- 1/4 cup (60 ml) milk (any type)
- Salt and pepper to taste
- 1 teaspoon olive oil
- 1 cup (about 50 g) fresh spinach leaves, washed

**INSTRUCTIONS:**

1. Combine the eggs, milk, salt, and pepper in a mid-sized mixing bowl. Use a whisk to blend these ingredients thoroughly until you achieve a uniform mixture.
2. Heat the olive oil in a nonstick skillet over medium heat. Introduce the spinach to the heated oil and sauté for 1-2 minutes, until the leaves have softened and reduced in volume.
3. Transfer the beaten eggs into the skillet containing the spinach. Continue cooking, using a spatula to gently move the eggs around the pan until they reach a mostly set consistency with a slight softness remaining, typically taking 3 to 5 minutes. Don't overcook.
4. Divide the scrambled eggs with spinach between two plates.

**Nutrition Per Serving:** Calories: 170 | Total Fat: 12g | Saturated Fat: 3g | Cholesterol: 300mg | Sodium: 140mg
Total Carbohydrate: 2g | Dietary Fiber: 1g | Sugars: 1g | Protein: 14g

## 18. Scrambled Eggs with Canned Peaches (2g fiber per serving)

**Yields:** 2 servings | **Prep Time:** 5 minutes | **Cook Time:** 5 minutes
**Fiber Content:** 2g per serving

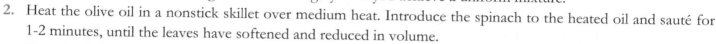

**Ingredients:**

- 4 large eggs
- 1/4 cup (60 ml) milk (any type)
- 1/4 teaspoon ground cinnamon
- Pinch of salt
- 1 tablespoon unsalted butter
- 1 (15-ounce) can sliced peaches in 100% juice, drained

**INSTRUCTIONS:**

1. Combine the eggs, milk, cinnamon, and salt in a moderately sized mixing bowl. Use a whisk to blend these ingredients thoroughly until you achieve a uniform mixture.
2. Melt the butter in a nonstick skillet over medium heat. Add the whisked egg mixture to the pan and continue cooking, gently moving the eggs around with a spatula until they're mostly set but retain a slight softness, typically taking 3 to 5 minutes. Don't overcook.
3. Divide the scrambled eggs between two plates. Top each serving with half of the drained sliced peaches.

**Nutrition Per Serving:** Calories: 230 | Total Fat: 14g | Saturated Fat: 5g | Cholesterol: 300mg | Sodium: 180mg
Total Carbohydrate: 16g | Dietary Fiber: 2g | Sugars: 12g | Protein: 14g

## 19. Chicken and Rice Soup with Carrots and Dill (4g fiber per serving)

**Yields:** 2 servings | **Prep Time:** 15 minutes | **Cook Time:** 30 minutes
**Fiber Content:** 4g per serving

**Ingredients:**

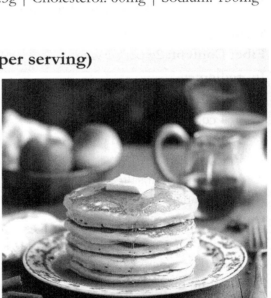

- 1 tablespoon olive oil
- 1 boneless, skinless chicken breast (about 6 ounces)
- 4 cups (960 ml) low-sodium chicken broth
- 1 cup (150 g) chopped carrots
- 1/2 cup (70 g) cooked white rice
- 1/4 cup chopped fresh dill
- Salt and pepper to taste

**INSTRUCTIONS:**

1. Warm the olive oil in a large pot or Dutch oven over medium heat. Add a dash of salt and pepper to both sides of the chicken breast. Place the seasoned chicken in the pot and cook for 5-7 minutes on each side. The chicken should develop a golden-brown color and be fully cooked inside.
2. Remove the cooked chicken breast from the pot and set it aside to cool slightly. Add the chicken broth, chopped carrots, and cooked rice to the pot. Heat the mixture until it begins to bubble, then reduce the heat and simmer gently for 15-20 minutes or until the carrots have softened.
3. While the soup simmers, shred the cooked chicken breast using two forks.
4. Add the shredded chicken and chopped fresh dill to the soup. Stir to combine and heat through. Season with salt and pepper to taste.

**Nutrition Per Serving:** Calories: 300 | Total Fat: 7g | Saturated Fat: 1.5g | Cholesterol: 60mg | Sodium: 150mg Total Carbohydrate: 35g | Dietary Fiber: 4g | Sugars: 4g | Protein: 30g

## 20 Applesauce Pancakes (4g fiber per serving)

**Yields:** About 6 pancakes (2 servings) | **Prep Time:** 5 minutes
**Cook Time:** 10-15 minutes | **Fiber Content:** 4g per serving

**Ingredients:**

- 1 cup (150g) all-purpose flour (or a gluten-free blend)
- 1 teaspoon baking powder
- 1/4 teaspoon salt
- 1 tablespoon granulated sugar (optional, for extra sweetness)
- 1 cup (240ml) unsweetened applesauce
- 1 cup (240ml) milk (or a plant-based alternative)
- 1 large egg
- 1 teaspoon vanilla extract

**INSTRUCTIONS:**

1. Mix the flour, sugar (if using), baking powder, and salt in a big bowl.
2. Mix the applesauce, milk, egg, and vanilla extract in another bowl.
3. mix the wet ingredients into the dry ingredients, whisking until just combined. Don't overmix; a few lumps are okay.
4. Heat a lightly greased skillet or griddle over medium heat. For each pancake, pour approximately 1/4 cup of batter onto the hot griddle. Cook for 2-3 minutes per side, or until golden brown and cooked through.

**Nutrition Per Serving (3 pancakes without toppings):** Calories: 320 | Total Fat: 6g | Saturated Fat: 2g Cholesterol: 55mg | Sodium: 500mg | Total Carbohydrate: 58g | Dietary Fiber: 4g | Sugars: 18g | Protein: 9g

## 21. Mashed Cauliflower with Herbs (4g fiber per serving)

**Yields:** 4 servings | **Prep Time:** 10 minutes | **Cook Time:** 15 minutes
**Fiber Content:** 4g per serving

**Ingredients:**

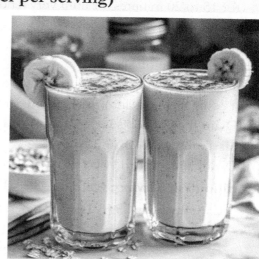

- 2 tablespoons fresh chives, finely chopped (for garnish)

**INSTRUCTIONS:**

1. Arrange the cauliflower florets and garlic cloves in a steaming basket above simmering water.
   Cover and steam for 10-12 minutes, or until very tender.
2. Once cooked, drain the cauliflower and garlic well, allowing them to steam dry for a few minutes.
3. Transfer the cauliflower and garlic to a food processor. Add milk, olive oil, dried thyme, dried rosemary, salt, and pepper.
4. Pulse the mixture until smooth and creamy, scraping down the sides as needed.
5. Taste and adjust seasoning if necessary.

**Nutrition Per Serving:** Calories: 120 | Total Fat: 8g | Saturated Fat: 1g | Cholesterol: 0mg | Sodium: 340mg
Total Carbohydrate: 11g | Dietary Fiber: 4g | Sugars: 4g | Protein: 4g

## 22. Banana Oatmeal Smoothie (4g fiber per serving)

**Yields:** 2 servings | **Prep Time:** 5 minutes | **Cook Time:** 0 minutes
**Fiber Content:** 4g per serving

**Ingredients:**

- 1 large ripe banana (about 6 ounces/170g), peeled and sliced
- 1/2 cup (40g) old-fashioned rolled oats
- 1 cup (240ml) unsweetened almond milk (or milk of choice)
- 1/4 cup (60g) plain Greek yogurt
- 1 tablespoon (15ml) honey
- 1/4 teaspoon (0.5g) ground cinnamon
- 1/2 cup (120ml) ice cubes
- 1/8 teaspoon (0.5g) vanilla extract (optional)

**INSTRUCTIONS:**

1. Place the components into your blender, following the sequence provided in the ingredient list.
2. Start blending at low speed, then gradually increase to high. Process the mixture for approximately 30 to 45 seconds, or until you achieve a silky, uniform consistency.
3. Add a little more milk if the smoothie is too thick. If it's too thin, add more ice or banana.

**Nutrition Per Serving:** Calories: 180 | Total Fat: 4g | Saturated Fat: 0.5g | Cholesterol: 5mg | Sodium: 80mg
Total Carbohydrate: 32g | Dietary Fiber: 4g | Sugars: 15g | Protein: 7g

## 23. Baked Cod with Mashed Sweet Potatoes (5g fiber per serving)

**Yields:** 2 servings | **Prep Time:** 15 minutes | **Cook Time:** 30-35 minutes | **Fiber Content:** 5g per serving

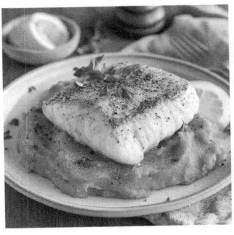

**Ingredients:**

**For the Cod:**

- 2 cod fillets (about 6 ounces/170g each)
- 1 tablespoon (15ml) olive oil
- 1/2 teaspoon (3g) salt
- 1/4 teaspoon (0.5g) black pepper
- 1 lemon, thinly sliced

**For the Mashed Sweet Potatoes:**

- 2 medium sweet potatoes (about 1 pound/450g total), peeled and cubed
- 2 tablespoons (30ml) unsweetened almond milk (or milk of choice)
- 1 tablespoon (14g) unsalted butter
- 1/4 teaspoon (1.5g) salt
- 1/8 teaspoon (0.25g) ground cinnamon (optional)

**INSTRUCTIONS:**

1. Set oven to 400°F (200°C).
2. Add the diced sweet potatoes to a medium-sized pot, cover with water, and bring to a boil. Simmer on low heat for 15 to 20 minutes, or until very tender.
3. While sweet potatoes cook, pat cod fillets dry with paper towels. Arrange the cod fillets in a suitable baking dish. Lightly coat each piece with olive oil, then sprinkle with a pinch of salt and freshly ground pepper. Top each fillet with lemon slices.
4. Transfer the prepared cod to the hot oven and cook for approximately 12 to 15 minutes. The fish is ready when it easily separates into flakes when gently pressed with a fork.
5. Drain the cooked sweet potatoes and return them to the pan. Add milk, butter, salt, and cinnamon (if using). Mash until smooth and creamy.
6. Divide the mashed sweet potatoes between two plates and top each with a baked cod fillet.

**Nutrition Per Serving:** Calories: 380 | Total Fat: 13g | Saturated Fat: 4g | Cholesterol: 70mg | Sodium: 820mg
Total Carbohydrate: 35g | Dietary Fiber: 5g | Sugars: 7g | Protein: 32g

## 24. Salmon Patties (No Breadcrumbs) (5g fiber per serving)

**Yields:** 2 servings | **Prep Time:** 15 minutes | **Cook Time:** 10 minutes | **Fiber Content:** 5g per serving

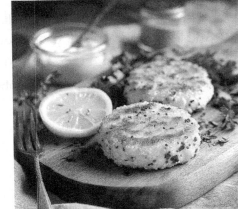

**Ingredients:**

- 1 (14-ounce / 400g) can salmon, drained and flaked
- 1/2 cup (50g) cooked quinoa, cooled
- 1/4 cup (30g) finely chopped onion
- 1 large egg, beaten
- 2 tablespoons (10g) chopped fresh parsley
- 1 tablespoon (7g) Dijon mustard
- 1/2 teaspoon (3g) salt
- 1/4 teaspoon (1g) black pepper
- 1 tablespoon (15 ml) olive oil, for cooking

**INSTRUCTIONS:**

1. In a medium bowl, combine the flaked salmon, cooked quinoa, chopped onion, beaten egg, chopped parsley, Dijon mustard, salt, and pepper. Gently mix until well combined.

2. Divide the salmon mixture into 2 equal portions. Form each half of the salmon mixture into a round, flattened cake approximately 1/2 inch (1.25 cm) in height.

3. Heat the olive oil in a large skillet over medium heat. Gently transfer the salmon cakes to the heated skillet and cook for approximately 4 to 5 minutes on each side, or until they develop a golden-brown crust and are fully cooked in the center.

4. Present the salmon patties warm, accompanied by your preferred side dishes, like a fresh green salad, gently steamed vegetables, or a dollop of unsweetened Greek yogurt.

**Nutrition Per Serving:** Calories: 380 | Total Fat: 20g | Saturated Fat: 3g | Cholesterol: 120mg | Sodium: 500mg Total Carbohydrate: 25g | Dietary Fiber: 5g | Sugars: 5g | Protein: 30g

## 25. Tofu and Vegetable Curry (Mild) (5g fiber per serving)

**Yields:** 2 servings | **Prep Time**: 15 minutes | **Cook Time**: 25 minutes | **Fiber Content**: 5g per serving

**Ingredients:**

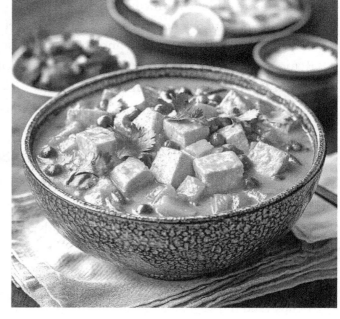

- 7 ounces (200g) firm tofu, pressed and cubed
- 1 tablespoon (15ml) olive oil
- 1/2 medium onion, finely chopped (about 1/2 cup/75g)
- 1 small carrot, diced (about 1/3 cup/50g)
- 1 small zucchini, diced (about 1/2 cup/75g)
- 1 clove garlic, minced
- 1 teaspoon (2g) mild curry powder
- 1/4 teaspoon (0.5g) ground turmeric
- 1/4 teaspoon (1.5g) salt
- 1/8 teaspoon (0.25g) black pepper
- 1 cup (240ml) low-sodium vegetable broth
- 1/4 cup (60ml) coconut milk
- 1/2 cup (75g) frozen peas
- 2 tablespoons (8g) fresh cilantro, chopped (optional)

**INSTRUCTIONS:**

1. Pat the cubed tofu dry with paper towels.
2. Heat olive oil in a large skillet over medium heat. Add onion and carrot, cooking for 5 minutes until softened. Add zucchini and garlic, cooking for another 2 minutes.
3. Stir in curry powder, turmeric, salt, and pepper. Cook for 1 minute until fragrant.
4. Add vegetable broth and coconut milk. Allow the mixture to reach a gentle bubbling state, then lower the heat and let it cook slowly for about 10 minutes.
5. Gently stir in the tofu cubes and frozen peas. Simmer for 5 minutes, or until peas are tender and tofu is heated through.
6. Divide the curry between two bowls. Garnish with fresh cilantro if desired.

**Nutrition Per Serving:** Calories: 250 | Total Fat: 16g | Saturated Fat: 5g | Cholesterol: 0mg | Sodium: 400mg Total Carbohydrate: 18g | Dietary Fiber: 5g | Sugars: 6g | Protein: 14g

## 26. Easy-to-Digest Oatmeal with Banana and Cinnamon (5g fiber per serving)

**Yields**: 2 servings | **Prep Time**: 5 minutes | **Cook Time**: 5-7 minutes | **Fiber Content**: 5g per serving

**Ingredients:**

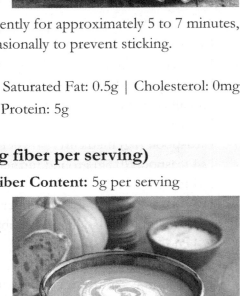

- 1 cup (48 g) rolled oats (not steel-cut)
- 2 cups (480 ml) water
- 1/4 teaspoon ground cinnamon
- Pinch of salt
- 1 ripe banana, mashed
- Optional toppings: a drizzle of honey or maple syrup, a sprinkle of chopped walnuts or pecans

**INSTRUCTIONS:**

1. In a medium saucepan, combine the rolled oats, water, cinnamon, and salt. Bring to a boil over medium heat.
2. After the mixture reaches a boil, lower the heat setting and let it bubble gently for approximately 5 to 7 minutes, or until the oats have softened and absorbed most of the liquid. Stir occasionally to prevent sticking.
3. Remove the oatmeal from the heat and stir in the mashed banana.

**Nutrition Per Serving (without toppings):** Calories: 200 | Total Fat: 3g | Saturated Fat: 0.5g | Cholesterol: 0mg Sodium: 5mg | Total Carbohydrate: 40g | Dietary Fiber: 5g | Sugars: 12g | Protein: 5g

## 27. Creamy Butternut Squash Soup (Strained) (5g fiber per serving)

**Yields**: 2 servings | **Prep Time**: 15 minutes | **Cook Time**: 30 minutes | **Fiber Content**: 5g per serving

**Ingredients:**

- 1 medium butternut squash (about 2 pounds), peeled, seeded, and cubed
- 1 tablespoon olive oil
- 1 medium onion, chopped
- 2 cloves garlic, minced
- 4 cups (960 ml) vegetable broth (or chicken broth)
- 1/2 teaspoon salt, or to taste
- 1/4 teaspoon black pepper, or to taste

**INSTRUCTIONS:**

1. Set your oven to heat up to 400°F (200°C). On a baking tray, combine the diced butternut squash with a drizzle of olive oil, a pinch of salt, and some ground pepper, ensuring all pieces are evenly coated. Roast for 25-30 minutes, or until tender.
2. As the butternut squash roasts, warm the olive oil in a spacious cooking vessel, such as a large pot or Dutch oven, set over medium heat. After adding the chopped onion to the heated oil, stir it occasionally for about 5 minutes, or until it softens and turns translucent. Next, incorporate the minced garlic into the pot with the softened onions. Continue cooking for another minute, or until the garlic releases its fragrant aroma.
3. Incorporate the oven-roasted butternut squash into the pot, then pour in the vegetable broth. Increase the heat until the mixture starts to bubble vigorously. Once boiling, lower the temperature and let it simmer gently for about 15 minutes, allowing the flavors to blend harmoniously.
4. Carefully transfer the soup to a blender (or use an immersion blender) and blend until completely smooth. Pour the blended soup through a fine-mesh strainer into a fresh pot to achieve an exceptionally smooth consistency.
5. Return the strained soup to the stovetop and heat through. Fine-tune the flavors by adding salt and pepper according to your preference.

**Nutrition Per Serving:** Calories: 250 | Total Fat: 6g | Saturated Fat: 1g | Cholesterol: 0mg | Sodium: 500mg
Total Carbohydrate: 48g | Dietary Fiber: 5g | Sugars: 8g | Protein: 5g

## 28. Ground Turkey and Rice Bowl (6g fiber per serving)

**Yields:** 2 servings | **Prep Time:** 15 minutes | **Cook Time:** 20 minutes | **Fiber Content:** 6g per serving
**Ingredients:**

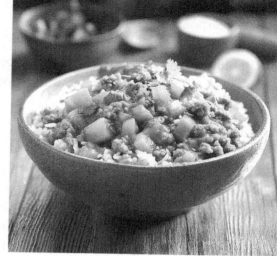

- 1 tablespoon (15 ml) olive oil
- 1/2 cup (80g) chopped onion
- 1/2 cup (80g) chopped green bell pepper
- 1 pound (450g) ground turkey (93% lean or higher)
- 1/2 teaspoon (1g) ground cumin
- 1/4 teaspoon (1g) salt
- 1/4 teaspoon (1g) black pepper
- 1 (14.5-ounce / 400g) can diced tomatoes, undrained
- 1/2 cup (120 ml) water
- 1 cup (185g) cooked brown rice
- 1/4 cup (10g) chopped fresh cilantro (optional)

**INSTRUCTIONS:**

1. Heat the olive oil in a large skillet over medium heat. Introduce the diced onion and green bell pepper to the heated oil. Cook, stirring occasionally, until they become tender, which usually takes around 5 minutes. Next, add the ground turkey to the pan. As it cooks, use a spoon to break it into smaller pieces, continuing until the meat has browned, which typically requires an additional 5 minutes.

2. Stir in the cumin, salt, and pepper. Continue cooking while stirring for 1 minute, allowing the spices to release their aromatic compounds. Stir in the diced tomatoes and water. Allow the mixture to reach a gentle bubbling point, then decrease the heat to its lowest setting. Place a lid on the pan and cook undisturbed for 10 minutes, allowing the flavors to blend harmoniously.

3. Divide the cooked brown rice between two bowls. Top each serving with the ground turkey mixture.

4. For an optional finishing touch, scatter a handful of finely minced cilantro over the top of the dish just before you bring it to the table.

**Nutrition Per Serving:** Calories: 370 | Total Fat: 14g | Saturated Fat: 3g | Cholesterol: 115mg | Sodium: 480mg
Total Carbohydrate: 42g | Dietary Fiber: 6g | Sugars: 6g | Protein: 32g

## 29. Baked Chicken Breast with Mashed Carrots (6g fiber per serving)

**Yields:** 2 servings | **Prep time:** 10 minutes | **Cook time:** 30 minutes
**Fiber Content:** 6g per serving

**Ingredients:**

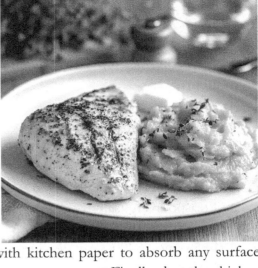

- 2 boneless, skinless chicken breasts (about 1 pound/450g total)
- 1 tablespoon (15 ml) olive oil
- 1/2 teaspoon (3g) salt
- 1/4 teaspoon (1g) black pepper
- 1 pound (450g) carrots, peeled and chopped
- 1/4 cup (60 ml) low-sodium chicken broth
- 1 tablespoon (15g) unsalted butter
- 1/4 teaspoon (0.5g) dried thyme

**INSTRUCTIONS:**

1. Preheat oven to 375°F (190°C). Gently blot the chicken breasts with kitchen paper to absorb any surface moisture. Next, drizzle a thin layer of olive oil over each piece, ensuring even coverage. Finally, dust the chicken with a pinch of salt and a few grinds of fresh black pepper.
2. Place the chicken breasts in a baking dish and bake for 25-30 minutes, or until cooked through and no longer pink inside. When placed inside the thickest area, an instant-read thermometer should read 165°F (74°C).
3. Boil salted water in a pot while the chicken bakes. Add the chopped carrots and cook until tender, about 10-12 minutes. Drain the carrots and return them to the pot.
4. Add the chicken broth, butter, and dried thyme to the pot with the carrots. With a potato masher or the tines of a fork, thoroughly mash the carrots, incorporating the added ingredients until you achieve a smooth, creamy consistency. Sample the mixture and enhance the flavor with extra salt and pepper as needed.
5. Serve the baked chicken breasts with a generous portion of mashed carrots.

**Nutrition Per Serving:** Calories: 350 | Total Fat: 15g | Saturated Fat: 4g | Cholesterol: 100mg | Sodium: 400mg
Total Carbohydrate: 30g | Dietary Fiber: 6g | Sugars: 10g | Protein: 35g

## 30. Poached Pears in Ginger Tea (6g fiber per serving)

**Yields:** 2 servings | **Prep Time:** 10 minutes | **Cook Time:** 20-25 minutes
**Fiber Content:** 6g per serving

**Ingredients:**

- 2 cups (480 ml) water
- 2 inches fresh ginger, peeled and thinly sliced
- 2 firm but ripe pears, such as Bosc or Anjou
- 2 tablespoons honey (or maple syrup)
- 1/2 teaspoon vanilla extract
- Pinch of ground cinnamon for garnish (optional)

**INSTRUCTIONS:**

1. In a saucepan, combine the water and ginger slices. Bring to a boil over medium-high heat. Lower the temperature and let the mixture gently bubble for about 10 minutes.
2. While the tea simmers, peel the pears, leaving the stems intact. Slice the pears down the middle, keeping the stems attached, then scoop out the central part containing the seeds using a small spoon or melon baller.
3. Add the pears to the simmering ginger tea. Increase heat to medium and bring to a gentle simmer. Cover the saucepan and cook for 15-20 minutes, or until the pears are tender when pierced with a fork.

4. Infuse with Honey and Vanilla: Stir in the honey (or maple syrup) and vanilla extract. Turn the heat down to its lowest setting and let the mixture gently cook for another 2 minutes, allowing the flavors to blend.

5. Carefully remove the pears from the cooking liquid using a slotted spoon. Divide them between two serving bowls. If you like, dust the top of each serving with a small amount of ground cinnamon for added flavor. Serve warm or chilled.

**Nutrition Per Serving:** Calories: 180 | Total Fat: 0g | Saturated Fat: 0g | Cholesterol: 0mg | Sodium: 10mg Total Carbohydrate: 45g | Dietary Fiber: 6g | Sugars: 30g | Protein: 1g

## 31. Baked Sweet Potato (7g fiber per serving)

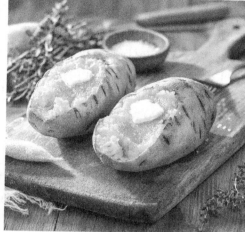

**Yields**: 2 servings | **Prep Time**: 5 minutes | **Cook Time**: 45-60 minutes
**Fiber Content:** 7g per serving

**Ingredients:**

- 2 medium sweet potatoes
- Olive oil or cooking spray

**INSTRUCTIONS:**

1. Set your oven to warm up to 400°F (200°C). Thoroughly wash the sweet potatoes, removing any dirt, then dry them off with a clean cloth or paper towel. With a fork, poke several holes into the skin of each sweet potato, ensuring they're evenly distributed.

2. Lightly rub the sweet potatoes with olive oil or spray them with cooking spray. Arrange the prepared sweet potatoes straight on the oven rack or a baking tray. Roast them for 45 to 60 minutes, until you can easily slide a fork into the flesh, indicating they're fully cooked.

**Nutrition Per Serving (without toppings):** Calories: 160 | Total Fat: 0g | Saturated Fat: 0g | Cholesterol: 0mg Sodium: 10mg | Total Carbohydrate: 37g | Dietary Fiber: 7g | Sugars: 13g | Protein: 3g

## 32. Creamy Coconut Chia Seed Pudding (8g fiber per serving)

**Yields**: 2 servings | **Prep Time**: 5 minutes | **Chill Time**: At least 2 hours (best overnight)
**Fiber Content:** 8g per serving

**Ingredients:**

- 1/2 cup (120ml) full-fat coconut milk
- 1/4 cup (60ml) unsweetened almond milk (or any milk alternative)
- 1/4 cup (40g) chia seeds
- 1 tablespoon maple syrup (or honey, to taste)
- 1/2 teaspoon vanilla extract
- Pinch of salt

**INSTRUCTIONS:**

1. In a medium-sized bowl, combine the coconut milk, almond milk, chia seeds, maple syrup, vanilla extract, and salt. Whisk the ingredients vigorously until you achieve a uniform mixture.

2. Place a cover over the bowl and let it rest in the refrigerator. Give the chia seeds at least 2 hours to absorb the liquid and plump up, but an overnight chill is best for the ideal pudding consistency.

3. Just before dishing out, thoroughly mix the pudding to ensure a consistent texture throughout. Divide into two serving bowls and top with your favorite low-fiber fruits (like a small amount of peeled and cooked apple or pear) if desired.

**Nutrition Per Serving:** Calories: 200 | Total Fat: 17g | Saturated Fat: 14g | Cholesterol: 0mg | Sodium: 35mg Total Carbohydrate: 16g | Dietary Fiber: 8g | Sugars: 11g | Protein: 3g

### 33. Well-Cooked Lentil Soup (Pureed) (18g fiber per serving)

**Yields:** 2 servings | **Prep Time:** 15 minutes | **Cook Time:** 40 minutes | **Fiber Content:** 18g per serving

**Ingredients:**

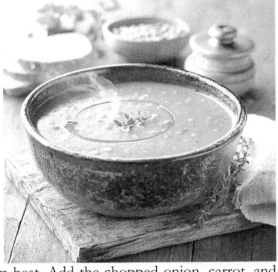

- 1 tablespoon (15ml) olive oil
- 1/2 cup (100g) chopped yellow onion
- 1/2 cup (70g) chopped carrot
- 1/2 cup (70g) chopped celery
- 1 teaspoon (2g) ground cumin
- 1/2 teaspoon (1g) dried thyme
- 1/4 teaspoon (1g) salt
- 1/4 teaspoon (1g) black pepper
- 1 cup (200g) brown lentils, rinsed
- 4 cups (960ml) low-sodium vegetable broth
- 1/2 cup (120ml) water

**INSTRUCTIONS:**

1. Warm the olive oil in a spacious pot or Dutch oven over medium heat. Add the chopped onion, carrot, and celery, and cook until softened about 5-7 minutes.
2. Stir in the ground cumin, dried thyme, salt, and pepper. Cook for 1 minute more, stirring constantly. Add the rinsed lentils and cook for 1 minute, stirring to coat.
3. Add the vegetable broth and water to the pot. Allow the mixture to reach a gentle boil, then lower the heat, cover the pot, and simmer for 30 minutes, or until the lentils become quite soft.
4. Cautiously pour the soup into a blender (or utilize an immersion blender) and blend until it becomes smooth. If the soup appears overly thick, add a small amount of water or broth to attain your preferred consistency.
5. Ladle the pureed lentil soup into bowls and serve hot.

**Nutrition Per Serving:** Calories: 320 | Total Fat: 7g | Saturated Fat: 1g | Cholesterol: 0mg | Sodium: 200mg
Total Carbohydrate: 50g | Dietary Fiber: 18g | Sugars: 5g | Protein: 20g

### Embracing A High-Fiber Lifestyle for Gut Health

The hidden hero of digestive health is fiber, particularly for people with diverticulosis. While a low-fiber diet may be necessary during acute flare-ups, transitioning to and maintaining a high-fiber diet is crucial for long-term gut health and preventing future complications.

## Why Fiber Matters:

1. Fiber adds bulk to your digestive system, which helps soften and ease waste passage. This reduces strain on your colon, potentially preventing the formation of new diverticula.
2. A high-fiber diet helps prevent constipation, which can exacerbate diverticulosis symptoms.
3. Certain types of fiber (prebiotics) nourish the good bacteria in your gut, promoting a healthy microbiome.
4. Foods high in fiber are typically more filling, which can help with weight management.

## Types of Fiber:

1. Soluble Fiber: Dissolves in water, forming a gel-like substance. It assists in controlling blood sugar and lowering cholesterol.
2. Fiber can be found in various food sources, including oats, barley, nuts, seeds, beans, lentils, peas, and many fruits and vegetables.
3. Insoluble Fiber: Doesn't dissolve in water. It makes the stool more substantial and facilitates the faster passage of food through the intestines and stomach.

Insoluble fiber can be found in various food sources, including whole grains, wheat bran, nuts, seeds, and the skins of many fruits and vegetables.

## Gradually Increasing Fiber Intake:

It's important to increase your fiber intake slowly to avoid discomfort. Start by adding 5 grams of fiber daily and gradually work up to the recommended amount over several weeks.

## Recommended Daily Fiber Intake: Women: 25 grams, Men: 38 grams

## Tips for Embracing a High-Fiber Diet:

1. Choose high-fiber breakfast options like oatmeal, bran cereal, or whole-grain toast.
2. Opt for fiber-rich snacks such as fresh fruits, vegetables with hummus, or a small handful of nuts.
3. Replace refined grains with whole grains in your meals. Think brown rice instead of white, whole-wheat pasta instead of regular.
4. Incorporate beans, lentils, and peas into your meals. They're excellent sources of both fiber and protein.
5. Try to fill half of your plate with fruits and vegetables at every meal.
6. When appropriate, eat the skins of fruits and vegetables, as they contain a significant amount of fiber.
7. Drink plenty of water as you increase your fiber intake to help it move through your digestive system.

Remember, everyone's digestive system is unique. If you experience discomfort as you increase your fiber intake, slow down and consult with your healthcare provider. They can provide personalized advice on how to best incorporate more fiber into your diet while managing your diverticulosis.

By embracing a high-fiber lifestyle, you're managing diverticulosis and promoting overall gut health and well-being. The recipes in this section are designed to help you easily and deliciously incorporate more fiber into your daily meals.

## 34. High-Fiber Berry Blast Smoothie

**Yields:** 2 servings | **Prep time:** 5 minutes

**Ingredients:**

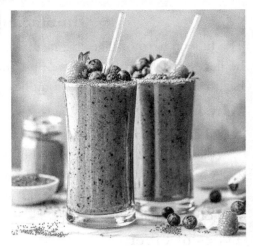

- 1 cup (150g) frozen mixed berries (strawberries, raspberries, blueberries)
- 1 ripe banana, sliced and frozen
- 1/2 cup (120ml) unsweetened almond milk (or milk of choice)
- 1/4 cup (60g) plain Greek yogurt
- 1 tablespoon (10g) chia seeds
- 1 tablespoon (17g) almond butter (or nut butter of choice)
- 1/2 teaspoon (2g) ground flaxseed

**INSTRUCTIONS:**

1. Combine all ingredients in a high-powered blender and blend until smooth and creamy. If necessary, incorporate additional almond milk, one tablespoon at a time, to achieve your preferred consistency.
2. Distribute the mixture between two glasses and consume promptly.

**Nutrition Per Serving:** Calories: 280 | Total Fat: 10g | Saturated Fat: 2g | Cholesterol: 5mg | Sodium: 50mg

Total Carbohydrate: 45g | Dietary Fiber: 12g | Sugars: 25g | Protein: 15g

## 35. Overnight Oats with Berries and Nuts

**Yields:** 2 servings | **Prep Time:** 5 minutes

**Ingredients:**

- 1 cup (100g) rolled oats (not instant)
- 1 cup (240ml) unsweetened almond milk (or milk of choice)
- 1/2 cup (70g) mixed berries (fresh or frozen)
- 1/4 cup (30g) chopped walnuts (or nuts of choice)
- 2 tablespoons (14g) chia seeds
- 1 tablespoon (15ml) maple syrup (optional, to taste)
- 1/2 teaspoon vanilla extract

**INSTRUCTIONS:**

1. In a moderately sized bowl, mix the rolled oats, almond milk, berries, walnuts, chia seeds, maple syrup (if desired), and vanilla extract.
2. Divide the mixture evenly between two jars or containers with lids. Secure the lids firmly and place the jars in the refrigerator for at least 2 hours, though leaving them overnight is ideal.
3. Enjoy cold straight from the refrigerator.

**Nutrition Per Serving:** Calories: 310 | Total Fat: 12g | Saturated Fat: 1g | Cholesterol: 0mg | Sodium: 10mg

Total Carbohydrate: 50g | Dietary Fiber: 10g | Sugars: 16g | Protein: 8g

## 36. Spinach and Feta Egg White Omelet

**Yields**: 2 servings | **Prep time**: 5 minutes | **Cook time**: 5 minutes

**Ingredients:**

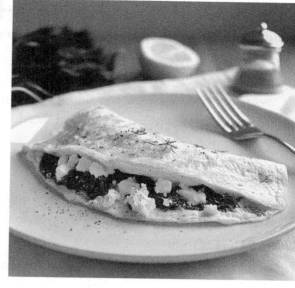

- 4 large egg whites
- 1/4 cup (60ml) water
- 1/4 teaspoon salt
- 1/4 teaspoon black pepper
- 1 tablespoon (14g) unsalted butter
- 1/2 cup (75g) chopped spinach, fresh or frozen (thawed and squeezed dry)
- 1/4 cup (60g) crumbled feta cheese
- 1 tablespoon (7g) chopped fresh dill (optional)

**INSTRUCTIONS:**

1. In a moderately sized bowl, use a whisk to blend the egg whites, water, salt, and pepper until the mixture becomes airy and foamy.
2. Heat the butter in a nonstick skillet over medium heat. Introduce the spinach to the pan and cook, stirring often, until it softens and shrinks, which typically takes around 2 minutes.
3. Pour the egg white mixture into the skillet and spread evenly. Cook for 3–4 minutes, or until the omelet is set and has a light golden bottom, lifting the edges regularly to allow the raw egg to flow below.
4. Sprinkle the feta cheese and dill (if using) over half of the omelet.
5. Carefully fold the unfilled half of the omelet over the filling. Gently transfer the omelet to a plate and present it for immediate consumption.

**Nutrition Per Serving:** Calories: 150 | Total Fat: 8g | Saturated Fat: 4g | Cholesterol: 10mg | Sodium: 400mg
Total Carbohydrate: 3g | Dietary Fiber: 1g | Sugars: 1g | Protein: 16g

## 37. Peach and Ginger Smoothie

**Yields**: 2 servings | **Prep time**: 5 minutes

**Ingredients:**

- 1 cup (150g) peeled and diced peaches (fresh or frozen)
- 1/2 cup (120ml) unsweetened almond milk (or milk of choice)
- 1/2 cup (120g) plain Greek yogurt
- 1 tablespoon (20g) honey (optional, to taste)
- 1/2 inch piece of fresh ginger, peeled and grated
- Pinch of ground cinnamon

**INSTRUCTIONS:**

1. Place all the listed ingredients into a blender and process until the mixture achieves a smooth and velvety consistency.
2. Should the smoothie appear overly thick, gradually incorporate additional almond milk until you achieve your preferred consistency.

**Nutrition Per Serving:** Calories: 180 | Total Fat: 3g | Saturated Fat: 1.5g | Cholesterol: 5mg | Sodium: 45mg
Total Carbohydrate: 35g | Dietary Fiber: 3g | Sugars: 25g | Protein: 8g

# 38. Apple Cinnamon Oatmeal with Flaxseed

**Yields**: 2 servings | **Prep time**: 5 minutes | **Cook time**: 5 minutes

**Ingredients:**

- 1 cup (80g) rolled oats (not instant)
- 2 cups (480ml) unsweetened almond milk (or milk of choice)
- 1 medium apple, peeled, cored, and diced
- 1 tablespoon (10g) ground flaxseed
- 1 teaspoon ground cinnamon
- 1/4 teaspoon ground nutmeg
- 2 tablespoons (14g) chopped walnuts (optional, for topping)
- 2 tablespoons (30ml) maple syrup (optional, to taste)

**INSTRUCTIONS:**

1. In a moderately sized saucepan, mix the oats, almond milk, diced apple, flaxseed, cinnamon, and nutmeg.
2. Bring the mixture to a boil over medium heat, then reduce heat to low and simmer for 5 minutes, or until the oats are cooked through and the liquid has been absorbed, stirring occasionally.
3. Distribute the oatmeal evenly between two bowls. Garnish each serving with a sprinkling of chopped walnuts and a light drizzle of maple syrup.

**Nutrition Per Serving:** Calories: 290 | Total Fat: 10g | Saturated Fat: 1g | Cholesterol: 0mg | Sodium: 10mg
Total Carbohydrate: 45g | Dietary Fiber: 10g | Sugars: 10g (excluding optional maple syrup) | Protein: 8g

# 39. Greek Yogurt Parfait with Berries and Granola

**Yields**: 2 servings | **Prep Time**: 10 minutes | **Cook Time**: 0 minutes

**Ingredients:**

- 1 cup (245g) plain Greek yogurt
- 1 tablespoon (21g) honey
- 1/4 teaspoon (1.25ml) vanilla extract
- 1 cup (150g) mixed berries (strawberries, blueberries, raspberries)
- 1/2 cup (50g) low-fat granola
- 2 teaspoons (10g) chia seeds

**INSTRUCTIONS:**

1. In a small bowl, mix the Greek yogurt, honey, and vanilla essence until thoroughly blended.
2. In two glasses or bowls, layer the ingredients as follows:
- 1/4 cup yogurt mixture
- 1/4 cup berries
- 2 tablespoons granola
3. Repeat the layers.
4. Top each parfait with 1 teaspoon of chia seeds.
5. Enjoy immediately or refrigerate for up to 2 hours before serving.

**Nutrition Per Serving:** Calories: 250 | Total Fat: 6g | Saturated Fat: 1g | Cholesterol: 5mg | Sodium: 50mg
Total Carbohydrate: 35g | Dietary Fiber: 6g | Sugars: 20g | Protein: 16g

## 40. Avocado Toast on Whole Grain Bread

**Yields:** 2 servings | **Prep Time:** 10 minutes | **Cook Time:** 5 minutes

**Ingredients:**

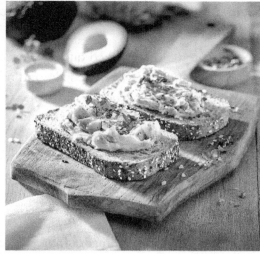

- 2 slices whole grain bread (about 2 ounces/56g each)
- 1 ripe avocado (about 5 ounces/150g)
- 1 tablespoon (15ml) fresh lemon juice
- 1/4 teaspoon (1.5g) salt
- 1/8 teaspoon (0.25g) black pepper
- 1/4 teaspoon (0.5g) red pepper flakes (optional)
- 2 teaspoons (10ml) extra virgin olive oil
- 2 tablespoons (10g) microgreens or sprouts (optional)

### INSTRUCTIONS:

1. Toast the whole grain bread slices until golden brown and crispy.
2. Remove the pit from the avocado, cut it in half, and scoop the flesh into a small bowl. Add lemon juice, salt, and pepper. Mash with a fork until slightly chunky.
3. Spread the mashed avocado evenly on the toasted bread slices.
4. Sprinkle red pepper flakes over the avocado if using. Drizzle each slice with 1 teaspoon of olive oil.

**Nutrition Per Serving:** Calories: 250 | Total Fat: 18g | Saturated Fat: 3g | Cholesterol: 0mg | Sodium: 380mg

Total Carbohydrate: 22g | Dietary Fiber: 8g | Sugars: 2g | Protein: 6g

## 41. Pumpkin Spice Smoothie Bowl

**Yields:** 2 servings | **Prep Time:** 10 minutes | **Cook Time:** 0 minutes

**Ingredients:**

**For the Smoothie:**

- 1 cup (245g) canned pumpkin puree
- 1 frozen banana (about 4 ounces/113g), sliced
- 1/2 cup (120ml) unsweetened almond milk
- 1/4 cup (60g) plain Greek yogurt
- 1 tablespoon (21g) maple syrup
- 1 teaspoon (2g) pumpkin pie spice
- 1/2 teaspoon (2.5ml) vanilla extract

**For the Toppings (per serving):**

- 1 tablespoon (10g) pumpkin seeds
- 1 tablespoon (6g) chopped pecans
- 1 teaspoon (5g) chia seeds
- Sprinkle of ground cinnamon

### INSTRUCTIONS:

1. In a blender, combine pumpkin puree, frozen banana, almond milk, Greek yogurt, maple syrup, pumpkin pie spice, and vanilla extract. Blend until smooth and creamy.
2. If the smoothie is too thick, add a little more almond milk. If it's too thin, add more frozen banana.
3. Sprinkle each bowl with pumpkin seeds, chopped pecans, chia seeds, and a dash of cinnamon.

**Nutrition Per Serving:** Calories: 250 | Total Fat: 11g | Saturated Fat: 1.5g | Cholesterol: 5mg | Sodium: 80mg

Total Carbohydrate: 35g | Dietary Fiber: 8g | Sugars: 18g | Protein: 8g

## 42. Quinoa Breakfast Bowl with Fresh Fruit

**Yields:** 2 servings | **Prep Time:** 5 minutes | **Cook Time:** 15 minutes

**Ingredients:**

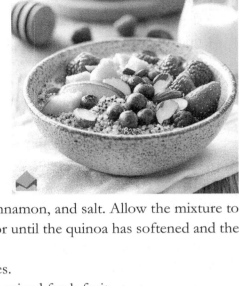

- 1/2 cup (85g) uncooked quinoa, rinsed
- 1 cup (240ml) unsweetened almond milk, plus more for serving
- 1 tablespoon (21g) honey or maple syrup
- 1/4 teaspoon (0.5g) ground cinnamon
- 1/8 teaspoon (0.25g) salt
- 1 cup (150g) mixed fresh fruit (e.g., berries, sliced peaches, diced mango)
- 2 tablespoons (14g) sliced almonds
- 2 teaspoons (10g) chia seeds

**INSTRUCTIONS:**

1. In a small saucepan, mix quinoa, almond milk, honey or maple syrup, cinnamon, and salt. Allow the mixture to boil, then lower the heat, cover the pan, and simmer for 12-15 minutes, or until the quinoa has softened and the liquid has been absorbed.
2. Remove from heat, fluff with a fork, and let stand, covered, for 5 minutes.
3. Divide the cooked quinoa between two bowls. Top each with half of the mixed fresh fruit.
4. Sprinkle each bowl with 1 tablespoon of sliced almonds and 1 teaspoon of chia seeds.
5. If desired, drizzle with additional almond milk and serve warm.

**Nutrition Per Serving:** Calories: 290 | Total Fat: 9g | Saturated Fat: 1g | Cholesterol: 0mg | Sodium: 160mg
Total Carbohydrate: 46g | Dietary Fiber: 7g | Sugars: 14g | Protein: 9g

## 43. Whole Grain Pancakes with Berry Compote

**Yields:** 2 servings (6 small pancakes) | **Prep Time:** 10 minutes | **Cook Time:** 15 minutes

**Ingredients:**

**For the Pancakes:**

- 3/4 cup (90g) whole wheat flour
- 1/4 cup (30g) rolled oats
- 1 teaspoon (5g) baking powder
- 1/4 teaspoon (1.5g) salt
- 1 cup (240ml) unsweetened almond milk
- 1 large egg
- 1 tablespoon (15ml) olive oil
- 1 tablespoon (21g) honey
- 1/2 teaspoon (2.5ml) vanilla extract

**For the Berry Compote:**

- 1 cup (150g) mixed berries (fresh or frozen)
- 2 tablespoons (30ml) water
- 1 tablespoon (21g) honey

**INSTRUCTIONS:**

1. In a large bowl, whisk together flour, oats, baking powder, and salt. In another bowl, mix almond milk, egg, olive oil, honey, and vanilla. Pour wet ingredients into dry and stir until just combined.
2. Heat a non-stick skillet or griddle over medium heat. Pour about 1/4 cup batter for each pancake. Cook for 2-3 minutes until bubbles form on the surface, then flip and cook for another 1-2 minutes.

3. While pancakes cook, combine berries, water, and honey in a small saucepan. Bring to a simmer over medium heat, stirring occasionally, until the sauce thickens and the berries break down, about 5 to 7 minutes.
4. Divide pancakes between two plates and top with warm berry compote.

**Nutrition Per Serving:** Calories: 380 | Total Fat: 12g | Saturated Fat: 2g | Cholesterol: 95mg | Sodium: 450mg Total Carbohydrate: 60g | Dietary Fiber: 8g | Sugars: 22g | Protein: 12g

## 44. Baked Oatmeal with Apples and Walnuts

**Yields:** 2 servings | **Prep Time:** 10 minutes | **Cook Time:** 25-30 minutes

**Ingredients:**

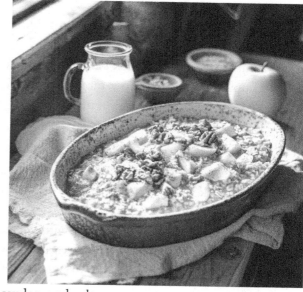

- 1 cup (90g) old-fashioned rolled oats
- 1/4 cup (30g) chopped walnuts
- 1 teaspoon (2g) ground cinnamon
- 1/4 teaspoon (1g) baking powder
- 1/8 teaspoon (0.75g) salt
- 1 cup (240ml) unsweetened almond milk
- 1 large egg
- 2 tablespoons (42g) maple syrup
- 1 teaspoon (5ml) vanilla extract
- 1 medium apple (about 6 ounces/170g), cored and diced
- 1 tablespoon (14g) unsalted butter, melted (optional)

**INSTRUCTIONS:**

1. Set oven to 375°F (190°C). Grease a 1-quart baking dish.
2. In a bowl, combine oats, half the walnuts, cinnamon, baking powder, and salt.
3. Almond milk, egg, maple syrup, and vanilla extract should all be combined in a separate bowl.
4. Stir the wet ingredients into the dry ingredients. Fold in half of the diced apple. Fill the baking dish with the mixture. Top with remaining apple and walnuts.
5. Drizzle with melted butter if using. Bake for 25-30 minutes, until the top is golden and the oatmeal is set.

**Nutrition Per Serving:** Calories: 340 | Total Fat: 16g | Saturated Fat: 3g | Cholesterol: 95mg | Sodium: 220mg Total Carbohydrate: 43g | Dietary Fiber: 7g | Sugars: 18g | Protein: 9g

# 45. Breakfast Burrito with Whole Wheat Tortilla

**Yields**: 2 servings | **Prep Time**: 10 minutes | **Cook Time**: 10 minutes

**Ingredients:**

- 2 large whole wheat tortillas (about 8 inches/20cm in diameter)
- 4 large eggs
- 2 tablespoons (30ml) unsweetened almond milk
- 1/4 teaspoon (1.5g) salt
- 1/8 teaspoon (0.25g) black pepper
- 1 tablespoon (15ml) olive oil
- 1/2 cup (75g) diced bell peppers (any color)
- 1/4 cup (40g) diced onion
- 1/2 cup (80g) canned black beans, rinsed and drained
- 1/4 cup (30g) shredded low-fat cheddar cheese
- 1/4 cup (60g) plain Greek yogurt
- 2 tablespoons (30g) mild salsa

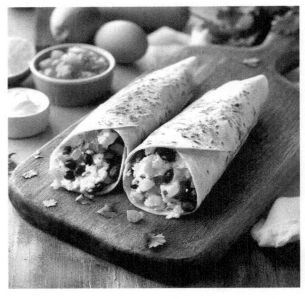

**INSTRUCTIONS:**

1. In a bowl, whisk together eggs, almond milk, salt, and pepper.
2. In a nonstick skillet, warm the olive oil over medium heat. Add bell peppers and onion, cooking until softened, about 3-4 minutes.
3. Add the egg mixture to the skillet with vegetables. Cook, stirring gently, until eggs are set but still moist.
4. In another skillet or on a griddle, warm the whole wheat tortillas for about 30 seconds on each side.
5. Divide the egg mixture between the two tortillas. Top each with half of the black beans, cheese, Greek yogurt, and salsa.
6. Fold in the sides of each tortilla and roll up from the bottom.

**Nutrition Per Serving:** Calories: 420 | Total Fat: 22g | Saturated Fat: 6g | Cholesterol: 380mg | Sodium: 780mg
Total Carbohydrate: 35g | Dietary Fiber: 8g | Sugars: 4g | Protein: 25g

# 46. Whole Grain English Muffin with Egg and Spinach

**Yields**: 2 servings | **Prep Time**: 5 minutes | **Cook Time**: 10 minutes

**Ingredients:**

- 2 whole-grain English muffins
- 2 large eggs
- 1 cup (30g) fresh baby spinach
- 2 teaspoons (10ml) olive oil, divided
- 2 tablespoons (30g) low-fat cream cheese
- Salt and pepper to taste
- 1/4 teaspoon (0.5g) dried oregano (optional)

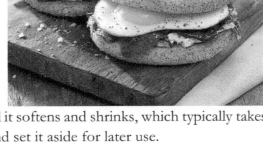

**INSTRUCTIONS:**

1. Split the English muffins and toast them until lightly golden.
2. Warm 1 teaspoon of olive oil in a small pan over medium heat. Introduce the spinach to the pan and cook, stirring occasionally, until it softens and shrinks, which typically takes about 1-2 minutes. Once done, transfer the spinach from the pan and set it aside for later use.
3. In the same pan, add the remaining teaspoon of olive oil over medium heat. Crack the eggs into the pan and cook to your preferred doneness (about 2-3 minutes for over-easy, 3-4 minutes for over-medium). Season with salt and pepper to taste.

4. On the bottom half of each English muffin, spread 1 tablespoon of cream cheese.
5. Top with the wilted spinach, dividing it equally between the two muffins.
6. Place a cooked egg on top of the spinach on each muffin.
7. Sprinkle with dried oregano if using. Top with the other half of the English muffin.

**Nutrition Per Serving:** Calories: 280 | Total Fat: 13g | Saturated Fat: 4g | Cholesterol: 195mg | Sodium: 350mg
Total Carbohydrate: 28g | Dietary Fiber: 5g | Sugars: 3g | Protein: 15g

## 47. Buckwheat Porridge with Cinnamon and Pear

**Yields**: 2 servings | **Prep Time**: 5 minutes | **Cook Time**: 15 minutes
**Ingredients:**

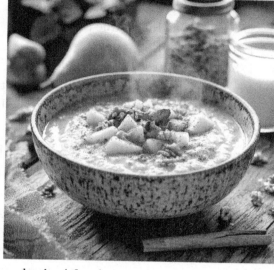

- 1/2 cup (85g) raw buckwheat groats
- 1 1/2 cups (360ml) unsweetened almond milk
- 1/4 teaspoon (1.5g) salt
- 1 teaspoon (2g) ground cinnamon
- 2 tablespoons (42g) maple syrup
- 1 medium ripe pear (about 6 ounces/170g), cored and diced
- 2 tablespoons (14g) chopped walnuts
- 1 tablespoon (15ml) coconut oil (optional)

## INSTRUCTIONS:

1. Buckwheat groats should be placed in a fine-mesh strainer and cleaned with cold water.
2. In a medium saucepan, combine rinsed buckwheat, almond milk, and salt. After bringing to a boil, lower the heat to a simmer and stir occasionally while the buckwheat absorbs most of the liquid. This process should take approximately 15 minutes.
3. Stir in cinnamon and maple syrup. Set the saucepan aside, away from the heat source, and let the mixture sit undisturbed for 5 minutes.
4. While the buckwheat is cooking, dice the pear and chop the walnuts.
5. Divide the porridge between two bowls. Top each with half of the diced pear and chopped walnuts. For those who prefer, finish each serving with a drizzle of coconut oil, using approximately 1/2 tablespoon per bowl.

**Nutrition Per Serving:** Calories: 310 | Total Fat: 11g | Saturated Fat: 4g | Cholesterol: 0mg | Sodium: 320mg
Total Carbohydrate: 50g | Dietary Fiber: 7g | Sugars: 20g | Protein: 7g

## 48. Tofu Scramble with Vegetables

**Yields:** 2 servings | **Prep Time:** 10 minutes | **Cook Time:** 15 minutes

**Ingredients:**

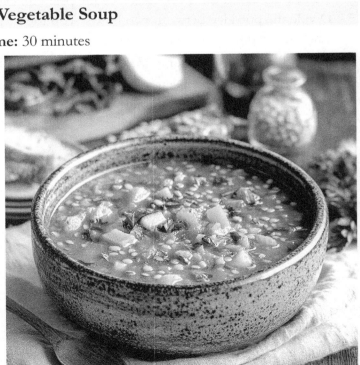

- 14 ounces (400g) firm tofu, drained and crumbled
- 1 tablespoon (15ml) olive oil
- 1/2 medium onion (about 2 ounces/60g), finely diced
- 1 small bell pepper (about 3 ounces/85g), diced
- 1 cup (30g) baby spinach
- 1/4 teaspoon (1.5g) turmeric powder
- 1/4 teaspoon (1.5g) garlic powder
- 1/4 teaspoon (1.5g) salt
- 1/8 teaspoon (0.25g) black pepper
- 1 tablespoon (15ml) nutritional yeast (optional, for a cheesy flavor)
- 2 tablespoons (8g) fresh chives, chopped

**INSTRUCTIONS:**

1. Drain the tofu and crumble it with your hands into bite-sized pieces.
2. Heat olive oil in a large non-stick skillet over medium heat. Add onion and bell pepper, cooking for 3-4 minutes until softened.
3. Introduce the crumbled tofu, turmeric, garlic powder, salt, and pepper to the skillet. Mix all ingredients together and allow them to cook for 5-6 minutes, stirring intermittently.
4. Add spinach and cook for another 1-2 minutes until wilted.
5. Stir in nutritional yeast if using. Taste and adjust seasonings if needed.

**Nutrition Per Serving:** Calories: 220 | Total Fat: 13g | Saturated Fat: 2g | Cholesterol: 0mg | Sodium: 380mg
Total Carbohydrate: 10g | Dietary Fiber: 5g | Sugars: 3g | Protein: 20g

---

## 2. Hearty Soups & Salads

## 49. Lentil and Vegetable Soup

**Yields:** 2 servings | **Prep Time:** 15 minutes | **Cook Time:** 30 minutes

**Ingredients:**

- 1/2 cup (100g) dried green or brown lentils, rinsed
- 2 tablespoons (30ml) olive oil
- 1 small onion (about 2 ounces/60g), diced
- 1 medium carrot (about 2 ounces/60g), diced
- 1 celery stalk (about 1 ounce/30g), diced
- 1 clove garlic, minced
- 1 small zucchini (about 4 ounces/113g), diced
- 1 14-ounce (400g) can diced tomatoes
- 3 cups (720ml) low-sodium vegetable broth
- 1 teaspoon (2g) dried thyme
- 1/2 teaspoon (1g) dried oregano
- 1/4 teaspoon (1.5g) salt
- 1/8 teaspoon (0.25g) black pepper
- 1 cup (30g) baby spinach
- 1 tablespoon (15ml) lemon juice
- 2 tablespoons (8g) fresh parsley, chopped

## INSTRUCTIONS:

1. Heat olive oil in a large pot over medium heat. Add onion, carrot, and celery. Cook for 5 minutes until softened.
2. Stir in garlic and cook for another minute until fragrant.
3. Add lentils, zucchini, diced tomatoes, vegetable broth, thyme, oregano, salt, and pepper. Bring to a boil.
4. Lentils should be soft after 25 to 30 minutes of simmering, covered, and low heat.
5. Stir in spinach and lemon juice. Cook the spinach for 2-3 minutes, or until it wilts.
6. Divide soup between two bowls and garnish with fresh parsley.

**Nutrition Per Serving:** Calories: 320 | Total Fat: 15g | Saturated Fat: 2g | Cholesterol: 0mg | Sodium: 580mg
Total Carbohydrate: 40g | Dietary Fiber: 16g | Sugars: 10g | Protein: 14g

## 50. Roasted Chickpea and Quinoa Salad

**Yields:** 2 servings | **Prep Time:** 15 minutes | **Cook Time:** 25 minutes

**Ingredients:**

**For the Roasted Chickpeas:**

- 1 15-ounce (425g) can chickpeas, drained, rinsed, and patted dry
- 1 tablespoon (15ml) olive oil
- 1/4 teaspoon (1.5g) salt
- 1/4 teaspoon (0.5g) paprika

**For the Salad:**

- 1/2 cup (85g) uncooked quinoa, rinsed
- 1 cup (240ml) water
- 2 cups (60g) mixed salad greens
- 1 small cucumber (about 4 ounces/113g), diced
- 1 medium tomato (about 4 ounces/113g), diced
- 1/4 red onion (about 1 ounce/28g), thinly sliced

**For the Dressing:**

- 2 tablespoons (30ml) extra virgin olive oil
- 1 tablespoon (15ml) lemon juice
- 1 teaspoon (5g) Dijon mustard
- 1/4 teaspoon (1.5g) salt
- 1/8 teaspoon (0.25g) black pepper

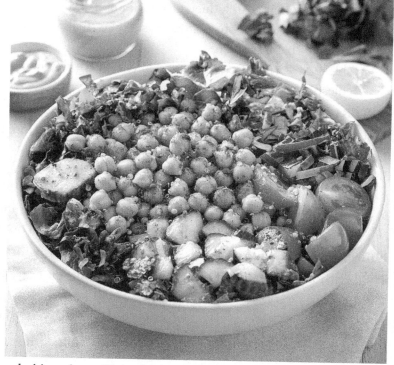

## INSTRUCTIONS:

1. Set oven to 400°F (200°C).
2. Toss chickpeas with olive oil, salt, and paprika on a baking sheet. Place in the oven and cook for 20-25 minutes, pausing halfway through to shake the pan gently to ensure even cooking. Continue roasting until the chickpeas achieve a crispy texture.
3. While chickpeas are roasting, combine quinoa and water in a saucepan. Allow the mixture to boil, then lower the heat, cover the saucepan, and simmer gently for 15 minutes. After this time, remove the saucepan from the heat source and let it sit undisturbed with the lid still on for 5 minutes. Finally, use a fork to lightly separate and fluff the quinoa grains.
4. In a large bowl, combine salad greens, cucumber, tomato, and red onion.
5. Olive oil, lemon juice, Dijon mustard, salt, and pepper should all be combined in a small bowl. Add cooked quinoa and roasted chickpeas to the vegetable mixture. Pour over the dressing and toss lightly to mix.

**Nutrition Per Serving:** Calories: 450 | Total Fat: 24g | Saturated Fat: 3g | Cholesterol: 0mg | Sodium: 750mg
Total Carbohydrate: 50g | Dietary Fiber: 12g | Sugars: 6g | Protein: 15g

## 51. Minestrone Soup with Whole Wheat Pasta

**Yields**: 2 servings | **Prep Time**: 15 minutes | **Cook Time**: 30 minutes

**Ingredients:**

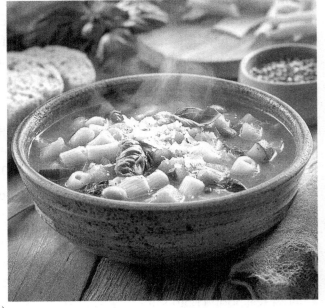

- 1 tablespoon (15ml) olive oil
- 1 small onion (about 2 ounces/60g), diced
- 1 medium carrot (about 2 ounces/60g), diced
- 1 celery stalk (about 1 ounce/30g), diced
- 1 clove garlic, minced
- 1 small zucchini (about 4 ounces/113g), diced
- 1 14-ounce (400g) can diced tomatoes
- 3 cups (720ml) low-sodium vegetable broth
- 1 cup (240ml) water
- 1 teaspoon (2g) dried oregano
- 1/2 teaspoon (1g) dried thyme
- 1/4 teaspoon (1.5g) salt
- 1/8 teaspoon (0.25g) black pepper
- 1 15-ounce (425g) can kidney beans, drained and rinsed
- 1/2 cup (50g) whole wheat small pasta (like shells or elbows)
- 1 cup (30g) baby spinach
- 2 tablespoons (10g) grated Parmesan cheese (optional)
- 2 tablespoons (8g) fresh basil, chopped

### INSTRUCTIONS:

1. Heat olive oil in a large pot over medium heat. Add onion, carrot, and celery. Cook for 5 minutes until softened.
2. Stir in garlic and cook for another minute until fragrant.
3. Add zucchini, diced tomatoes, vegetable broth, water, oregano, thyme, salt, and pepper. Bring to a boil.
4. Reduce heat to low, cover, and simmer for 15 minutes.
5. Add kidney beans and pasta. Simmer for another 8-10 minutes or until pasta is tender.
6. Stir in spinach and cook for 1-2 minutes until wilted. Top with Parmesan cheese (if using) and fresh basil.

**Nutrition Per Serving:** Calories: 360 | Total Fat: 9g | Saturated Fat: 2g | Cholesterol: 5mg | Sodium: 680mg
Total Carbohydrate: 58g | Dietary Fiber: 14g | Sugars: 12g | Protein: 17g

## 52. Greek Salad with Grilled Chicken

**Yields**: 2 servings | **Prep Time**: 15 minutes | **Cook Time**: 10 minutes

**Ingredients:**

**For the Chicken:**

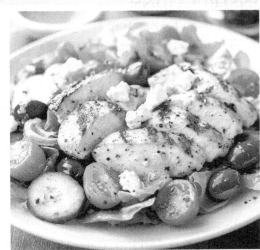

- 2 small boneless, skinless chicken breasts (about 4 ounces/113g each)
- 1 tablespoon (15ml) olive oil
- 1 teaspoon (2g) dried oregano
- 1/4 teaspoon (1.5g) salt
- 1/8 teaspoon (0.25g) black pepper

**For the Salad:**

- 4 cups (120g) chopped romaine lettuce
- 1 medium cucumber (about 8 ounces/226g), diced
- 1 cup (150g) cherry tomatoes, halved
- 1/2 small red onion (about 2 ounces/56g), thinly sliced

- 1/4 cup (35g) pitted Kalamata olives, halved
- 1/4 cup (30g) crumbled feta cheese

**For the Dressing:**
- 2 tablespoons (30ml) extra virgin olive oil
- 1 tablespoon (15ml) red wine vinegar
- 1/2 teaspoon (2.5g) Dijon mustard
- 1/4 teaspoon (1.5g) dried oregano
- 1/4 teaspoon (1.5g) salt
- 1/8 teaspoon (0.25g) black pepper

**INSTRUCTIONS:**
1. Season chicken breasts with salt, pepper, and oregano after brushing them with olive oil.
2. The internal temperature of the chicken should reach 165°F (74°C) after grilling it for 5–6 minutes on each side. Let rest for 5 minutes, then slice.
3. In a small bowl, whisk together all dressing ingredients.
4. In a large bowl, combine romaine lettuce, cucumber, tomatoes, red onion, and olives.
5. Add sliced chicken and crumbled feta to the salad. Pour over the dressing and toss lightly to mix.

**Nutrition Per Serving:** Calories: 400 | Total Fat: 28g | Saturated Fat: 6g | Cholesterol: 85mg | Sodium: 950mg Total Carbohydrate: 15g | Dietary Fiber: 5g | Sugars: 6g | Protein: 28g

## 53. Butternut Squash and Apple Soup

**Yields**: 2 servings | **Prep Time**: 15 minutes | **Cook Time**: 30 minutes

**Ingredients:**

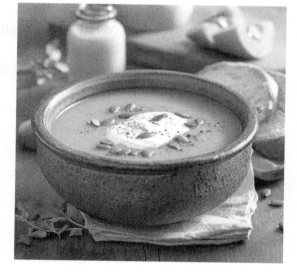

- 1 tablespoon (15ml) olive oil
- 1 small onion (about 2 ounces/60g), diced
- 1 medium apple (about 6 ounces/170g), peeled, cored, and diced
- 2 cups (300g) butternut squash, peeled and cubed
- 2 cups (480ml) low-sodium vegetable broth
- 1/4 teaspoon (0.5g) ground cinnamon
- 1/8 teaspoon (0.25g) ground nutmeg
- 1/4 teaspoon (1.5g) salt
- 1/8 teaspoon (0.25g) black pepper
- 1/4 cup (60ml) unsweetened almond milk
- 2 tablespoons (30g) plain Greek yogurt (optional, for garnish)
- 2 tablespoons (14g) pumpkin seeds (optional, for garnish)

**INSTRUCTIONS:**
1. Warm the olive oil in a spacious pot set over medium heat. Introduce the onion to the heated oil and sauté for approximately 3-4 minutes, or until the onion becomes tender and translucent.
2. Stir in diced apple and butternut squash. Cook for 5 minutes, stirring occasionally.
3. Pour in vegetable broth. Add cinnamon, nutmeg, salt, and pepper. Bring to a boil.
4. Turn the heat down to low, place a lid on the pot, and allow the mixture to simmer quietly for approximately 20 minutes. You'll know the squash is ready when it's extremely soft and yields easily to gentle pressure from a fork.
5. Remove from heat. Using an immersion blender, process the soup directly in the pot until it reaches a smooth consistency. Stir in almond milk. Taste and adjust seasonings if needed.

**Nutrition Per Serving:** Calories: 200 | Total Fat: 8g | Saturated Fat: 1g | Cholesterol: 0mg | Sodium: 420mg Total Carbohydrate: 32g | Dietary Fiber: 6g | Sugars: 12g | Protein: 4g

# 54. Spinach and Strawberry Salad with Poppy Seed Dressing

**Yields:** 2 servings | **Prep Time:** 15 minutes | **Cook Time:** 0 minutes

**Ingredients:**

**For the Salad:**

- 4 cups (120g) fresh baby spinach
- 1 cup (150g) fresh strawberries, hulled and sliced
- 1/4 cup (30g) sliced almonds, toasted
- 1/4 small red onion (about 1 ounce/28g), thinly sliced
- 2 ounces (56g) soft goat cheese, crumbled (optional)

**For the Poppy Seed Dressing:**

- 2 tablespoons (30ml) extra virgin olive oil
- 1 tablespoon (15ml) apple cider vinegar
- 1 teaspoon (5g) honey
- 1/2 teaspoon (2.5g) Dijon mustard
- 1/4 teaspoon (1.5g) poppy seeds
- 1/8 teaspoon (0.75g) salt
- Pinch of black pepper

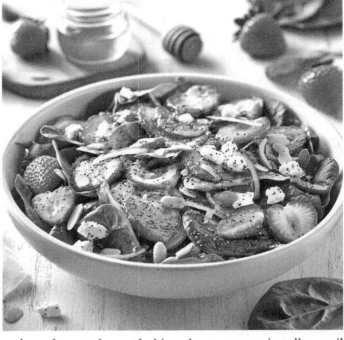

## INSTRUCTIONS:

1. Place a dry skillet over medium heat. Add the sliced almonds and toast them, shaking the pan occasionally, until they become lightly golden and emit a pleasant, nutty aroma. This process typically takes about 3-5 minutes. Once toasted, remove from heat and transfer to a cool plate to allow them to cool completely.

2. In a small mixing bowl, vigorously whisk together the olive oil, apple cider vinegar, honey, Dijon mustard, poppy seeds, salt, and pepper. Whisk energetically until all ingredients are fully incorporated and the dressing achieves a uniform, slightly thickened texture.

3. In a spacious salad bowl, gently toss the fresh spinach leaves, thinly sliced strawberries, and finely chopped red onion.

4. Pour the prepared poppy seed dressing evenly over the salad ingredients. Using salad tongs or two large spoons, delicately toss the mixture to ensure all components are lightly and uniformly coated with the dressing.

5. Divide the salad between two plates. Top each with toasted almonds and crumbled goat cheese, if using.

**Nutrition Per Serving:** Calories: 250 | Total Fat: 20g | Saturated Fat: 4g | Cholesterol: 10mg | Sodium: 280mg
Total Carbohydrate: 15g | Dietary Fiber: 5g | Sugars: 8g | Protein: 8g

# 55. Turkey and Bean Chili

**Yields**: 2 servings | **Prep Time**: 15 minutes | **Cook Time**: 30 minutes

## Ingredients:

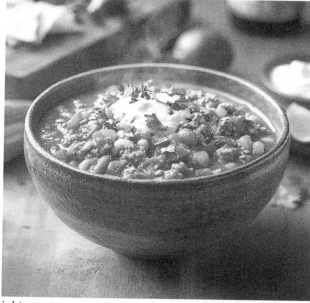

- 1/2 pound (225g) lean ground turkey
- 1 tablespoon (15ml) olive oil
- 1 small onion (about 2 ounces/60g), diced
- 1 small bell pepper (about 3 ounces/85g), diced
- 2 cloves garlic, minced
- 1 14-ounce (400g) can diced tomatoes
- 1 15-ounce (425g) can kidney beans, drained and rinsed
- 1 cup (240ml) low-sodium chicken broth
- 1 tablespoon (8g) chili powder
- 1 teaspoon (2g) ground cumin
- 1/2 teaspoon (1g) dried oregano
- 1/4 teaspoon (1.5g) salt
- 1/8 teaspoon (0.25g) black pepper
- 1/4 cup (30g) plain Greek yogurt (optional, for topping)
- 2 tablespoons (8g) fresh cilantro, chopped (optional, for garnish)

## INSTRUCTIONS:

1. In a large pot over medium heat, brown the ground turkey, using a wooden spoon to break it into small, even pieces as it cooks. Continue until the meat is fully cooked and no pink color remains. Remove from pot and set aside.
2. In the same pot, heat olive oil. Add onion and bell pepper, cooking for 5 minutes until softened.
3. Add the minced garlic and stir until fragrant, about 1 more minute.
4. Return cooked turkey to the pot. Add diced tomatoes, kidney beans, chicken broth, chili powder, cumin, oregano, salt, and pepper.
5. Increase the heat to high and allow the mixture to reach a rolling boil. Once boiling, promptly lower the heat to a gentle simmer. Place a lid on the pot and let it cook for 20 minutes, remembering to stir the contents every few minutes to prevent sticking.
6. Divide chili between two bowls. If desired, top each with a dollop of Greek yogurt and sprinkle with fresh cilantro.

**Nutrition Per Serving:** Calories: 420 | Total Fat: 15g | Saturated Fat: 3g | Cholesterol: 65mg | Sodium: 680mg
Total Carbohydrate: 40g | Dietary Fiber: 13g | Sugars: 8g | Protein: 35g

# 56. Kale and Roasted Vegetable Salad

**Yields**: 2 servings | **Prep Time**: 15 minutes | **Cook Time**: 25 minutes

## Ingredients:

### For the Roasted Vegetables:

- 1 cup (150g) butternut squash, peeled and cubed
- 1 cup (100g) Brussels sprouts, halved
- 1 small red onion (about 2 ounces/60g), cut into wedges
- 2 tablespoons (30ml) olive oil
- 1/4 teaspoon (1.5g) salt
- 1/8 teaspoon (0.25g) black pepper

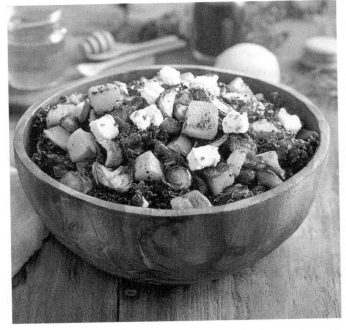

### For the Salad:

- 4 cups (120g) kale, stems removed and leaves chopped
- 1 tablespoon (15ml) lemon juice
- 1 teaspoon (5ml) olive oil
- Pinch of salt

### For the Dressing:

- 2 tablespoons (30ml) extra virgin olive oil
- 1 tablespoon (15ml) balsamic vinegar
- 1 teaspoon (5g) Dijon mustard
- 1 teaspoon (5g) honey
- 1/4 teaspoon (1.5g) salt
- 1/8 teaspoon (0.25g) black pepper

### Additional:

- 1/4 cup (30g) pumpkin seeds
- 2 ounces (56g) goat cheese, crumbled (optional)

## INSTRUCTIONS:

1. Set oven to 400°F (200°C).
2. On a baking sheet, toss together butternut squash, Brussels sprouts, and red onion with olive oil, salt, and pepper. Roast veggies for 20 to 25 minutes, stirring occasionally, or until they are soft and have a light brown color.
3. To soften the leaves, knead kale in a big bowl for approximately a minute with lemon juice, 1 teaspoon olive oil, and a pinch of salt.
4. In a small bowl, whisk together olive oil, balsamic vinegar, Dijon mustard, honey, salt, and pepper.
5. In a dry skillet over medium heat, toast pumpkin seeds until lightly golden and fragrant, about 2-3 minutes.
6. Add roasted vegetables to the bowl with kale. Drizzle the prepared dressing evenly over the salad ingredients, then use salad tongs or two large spoons to gently toss everything together, ensuring all components are lightly and uniformly coated with the dressing.
7. Divide the salad between two plates. Top each with toasted pumpkin seeds and crumbled goat cheese, if using.

**Nutrition Per Serving:** Calories: 420 | Total Fat: 32g | Saturated Fat: 6g | Cholesterol: 10mg | Sodium: 750mg

Total Carbohydrate: 30g | Dietary Fiber: 7g | Sugars: 10g | Protein: 12g

# 57. Carrot and Ginger Soup

**Yields**: 2 servings | **Prep Time**: 15 minutes | **Cook Time**: 25 minutes

## Ingredients:

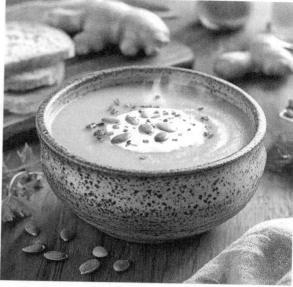

- 1 tablespoon (15ml) olive oil
- 1 small onion (about 2 ounces/60g), diced
- 2 cloves garlic, minced
- 1 tablespoon (6g) fresh ginger, grated
- 4 medium carrots (about 8 ounces/225g), peeled and chopped
- 2 cups (480ml) low-sodium vegetable broth
- 1/4 teaspoon (1.5g) salt
- 1/8 teaspoon (0.25g) black pepper
- 1/4 cup (60ml) unsweetened almond milk
- 2 tablespoons (30g) plain Greek yogurt (optional, for garnish)
- 2 teaspoons (6g) pumpkin seeds (optional, for garnish)
- Fresh chives, chopped (optional, for garnish)

## INSTRUCTIONS:

1. In a medium pot, heat olive oil over medium heat. Add the diced onion and sauté for 3-4 minutes, stirring occasionally, until it becomes translucent and soft. Incorporate the minced garlic and freshly grated ginger into the softened onions. Cook for 30-60 seconds, stirring frequently, until the garlic turns golden and the ginger becomes fragrant.

2. Add chopped carrots, vegetable broth, salt, and pepper. Increase the heat to high and allow the mixture to reach a rolling boil. Once boiling, promptly lower the heat to maintain a gentle simmer. Cover and simmer for 15-20 minutes, or until carrots are very tender.

3. Remove from heat. Carefully insert an immersion blender into the soup and blend, moving it around the pot, until the mixture reaches a smooth, creamy consistency. Alternatively, carefully transfer to a blender in batches.

4. Stir in almond milk. If the soup is too thick, add more broth or almond milk to reach desired consistency. Taste and adjust seasonings if needed.

5. Divide soup between two bowls. If desired, top each with a dollop of Greek yogurt, a sprinkle of pumpkin seeds, and chopped chives.

**Nutrition Per Serving:** Calories: 150 | Total Fat: 8g | Saturated Fat: 1g | Cholesterol: 0mg | Sodium: 480mg
Total Carbohydrate: 18g | Dietary Fiber: 4g | Sugars: 8g | Protein: 4g

## 58. Tabbouleh Salad with Quinoa

**Yields**: 2 servings | **Prep Time**: 20 minutes | **Cook Time**: 15 minutes (for quinoa) | **Chill Time**: 30 minutes

**Ingredients:**

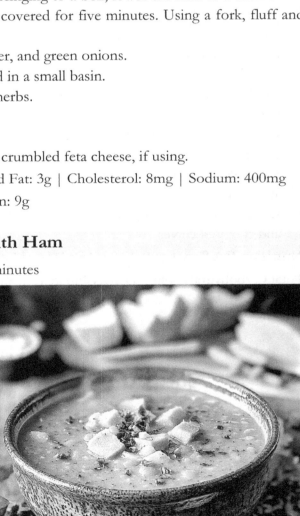

- 1/2 cup (85g) uncooked quinoa, rinsed
- 1 cup (240ml) water
- 2 cups (60g) fresh parsley, finely chopped
- 1/2 cup (15g) fresh mint leaves, finely chopped
- 1 medium tomato (about 4 ounces/113g), diced
- 1/2 English cucumber (about 4 ounces/113g), diced
- 2 green onions, thinly sliced
- 2 tablespoons (30ml) extra virgin olive oil
- 2 tablespoons (30ml) fresh lemon juice
- 1/4 teaspoon (1.5g) salt
- 1/8 teaspoon (0.25g) black pepper
- 1/4 cup (30g) crumbled feta cheese (optional)

**INSTRUCTIONS:**

1. Quinoa and water should be combined in a small pot. After bringing to a boil, lower the heat to a simmer for fifteen minutes while covered. Take off the heat and leave it covered for five minutes. Using a fork, fluff and allow to cool fully.
2. While quinoa is cooking, chop parsley, mint, tomato, cucumber, and green onions.
3. Olive oil, lemon juice, salt, and pepper should all be combined in a small basin.
4. In a large bowl, mix cooled quinoa, chopped vegetables, and herbs.
5. Pour the dressing over the salad and toss gently to combine.
6. Refrigerate for at least 30 minutes to allow flavors to meld.
7. Divide the salad between two plates. Before serving, top with crumbled feta cheese, if using.

**Nutrition Per Serving:** Calories: 300 | Total Fat: 18g | Saturated Fat: 3g | Cholesterol: 8mg | Sodium: 400mg
Total Carbohydrate: 30g | Dietary Fiber: 6g | Sugars: 3g | Protein: 9g

## 59. Split Pea Soup with Ham

**Yields**: 2 servings | **Prep Time**: 15 minutes | **Cook Time**: 45 minutes

**Ingredients:**

- 1 cup (200g) dried green split peas, rinsed and sorted
- 2 cups (480ml) low-sodium chicken broth
- 1 cup (240ml) water
- 1 tablespoon (15ml) olive oil
- 1 small onion (about 2 ounces/60g), diced
- 1 medium carrot (about 2 ounces/60g), diced
- 1 celery stalk (about 1 ounce/30g), diced
- 1 clove garlic, minced
- 4 ounces (113g) cooked ham, diced
- 1 bay leaf
- 1/4 teaspoon (0.5g) dried thyme
- 1/4 teaspoon (1.5g) salt
- 1/8 teaspoon (0.25g) black pepper
- 2 tablespoons (8g) fresh parsley, chopped (for garnish)

## INSTRUCTIONS:

1. In a large pot, heat olive oil over medium heat. Add onion, carrot, and celery. Cook for 5 minutes until softened. Add garlic and cook for another minute.
2. Stir in split peas, chicken broth, water, diced ham, bay leaf, thyme, salt, and pepper.
3. Bring to a boil, then reduce heat to low. Simmer, covered, stirring occasionally, for 40–45 minutes or until the soup has thickened and the peas are soft.
4. Take off the bay leaf. You may leave the soup as is for a chunkier soup or use an immersion blender to partially puree it for a creamier texture. Garnish with fresh parsley.

**Nutrition Per Serving:** Calories: 380 | Total Fat: 10g | Saturated Fat: 2g | Cholesterol: 25mg | Sodium: 850mg
Total Carbohydrate: 50g | Dietary Fiber: 20g | Sugars: 8g | Protein: 28g

## 60. Asian-Inspired Cabbage Salad

**Yields**: 2 servings | **Prep Time**: 20 minutes | **Chill Time**: 30 minutes (optional)

**Ingredients:**

**For the Salad:**

- 3 cups (225g) Napa cabbage, thinly sliced
- 1 cup (70g) red cabbage, thinly sliced
- 1 medium carrot (about 2 ounces/60g), julienned
- 1/2 red bell pepper (about 2 ounces/60g), thinly sliced
- 2 green onions, thinly sliced
- 1/4 cup (30g) unsalted peanuts, roughly chopped
- 2 tablespoons (8g) fresh cilantro, chopped

**For the Dressing:**

- 2 tablespoons (30ml) rice vinegar
- 1 tablespoon (15ml) low-sodium soy sauce
- 1 tablespoon (15ml) honey
- 1 tablespoon (15ml) sesame oil
- 1 teaspoon (5g) grated fresh ginger
- 1 small clove garlic, minced

## INSTRUCTIONS:

1. In a large bowl, combine Napa cabbage, red cabbage, carrot, bell pepper, and green onions.
2. Combine rice vinegar, soy sauce, honey, sesame oil, grated ginger, and chopped garlic in a small bowl.
3. Pour the dressing over the vegetables and toss well to combine.
4. If time allows, refrigerate the salad for 30 minutes to let the flavors meld.
5. Just before serving, add chopped peanuts and cilantro. Toss gently to combine.

**Nutrition Per Serving:** Calories: 220 | Total Fat: 14g | Saturated Fat: 2g | Cholesterol: 0mg | Sodium: 350mg
Total Carbohydrate: 22g | Dietary Fiber: 6g | Sugars: 13g | Protein: 6g

## 61. Tomato and Basil Soup with Whole Grain Croutons

**Yields:** 2 servings | **Prep Time:** 15 minutes | **Cook Time:** 30 minutes

**Ingredients:**

**For the Soup:**

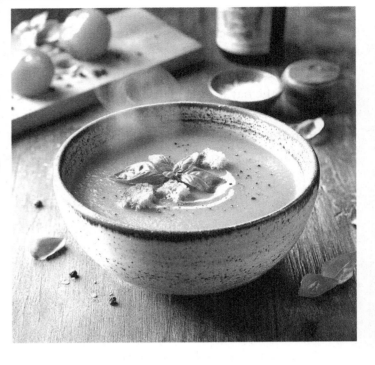

- 1 tablespoon (15ml) olive oil
- 1 small onion (about 2 ounces/60g), diced
- 2 cloves garlic, minced
- 1 28-ounce (800g) can whole peeled tomatoes
- 1 cup (240ml) low-sodium vegetable broth
- 1/4 cup (10g) fresh basil leaves, plus extra for garnish
- 1/4 teaspoon (1.5g) salt
- 1/8 teaspoon (0.25g) black pepper
- 2 tablespoons (30ml) heavy cream (optional)

**For the Whole Grain Croutons:**

- 2 slices whole grain bread, cut into 1/2-inch cubes
- 1 tablespoon (15ml) olive oil
- 1/4 teaspoon (0.5g) dried oregano
- 1/8 teaspoon (0.75g) salt

**INSTRUCTIONS:**

1. Preheat oven to 375°F (190°C). Mix salt, oregano, and olive oil with the bread cubes. Spread on a baking sheet and bake for 10-12 minutes, stirring halfway through, until golden and crisp. Set aside.
2. In a large pot, heat olive oil over medium heat. Add onion and simmer until softened, about 5 minutes. Add garlic and cook for another minute.
3. Pour in canned tomatoes with their juice, crushing them with your hands as you add them. Add vegetable broth, basil, salt, and pepper.
4. Bring to a boil, then reduce heat to low. Simmer for 20 minutes, stirring occasionally.

**Nutrition Per Serving:** Calories: 250 | Total Fat: 14g | Saturated Fat: 3g | Cholesterol: 10mg | Sodium: 650mg
Total Carbohydrate: 28g | Dietary Fiber: 6g | Sugars: 12g | Protein: 7g

## 62. Grilled Vegetable and Chickpea Salad

**Yields:** 2 servings | **Prep Time:** 15 minutes | **Cook Time:** 15 minutes

**Ingredients:**

**For the Salad:**

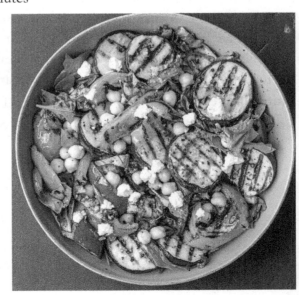

- 1 medium zucchini (about 6 ounces/170g), sliced lengthwise
- 1 small eggplant (about 6 ounces/170g), sliced into rounds
- 1 red bell pepper, cut into quarters
- 1 tablespoon (15ml) olive oil
- 1 15-ounce (425g) can chickpeas, drained and rinsed
- 2 cups (60g) mixed salad greens
- 1/4 cup (40g) crumbled feta cheese (optional)

**For the Dressing:**

- 2 tablespoons (30ml) extra virgin olive oil
- 1 tablespoon (15ml) balsamic vinegar
- 1 teaspoon (5g) Dijon mustard

- 1 small clove garlic, minced
- 1/4 teaspoon (1.5g) salt
- 1/8 teaspoon (0.25g) black pepper
- 1 teaspoon (1g) dried oregano

## INSTRUCTIONS:

1. Preheat grill or grill pan to medium-high heat.
2. Brush zucchini, eggplant, and bell pepper with olive oil. Grill for 3-4 minutes per side, until tender and lightly charred. Remove from grill and let cool slightly.
3. Mix olive oil, balsamic vinegar, Dijon mustard, minced garlic, salt, pepper, and dried oregano in a small bowl.
4. Once cooled, chop the grilled vegetables into bite-sized pieces.
5. In a large bowl, combine grilled vegetables, chickpeas, and mixed salad greens.
6. Pour the dressing over the salad and toss gently to combine. Top with crumbled feta cheese, if using.

**Nutrition Per Serving:** Calories: 380 | Total Fat: 22g | Saturated Fat: 4g | Cholesterol: 8mg | Sodium: 680mg Total Carbohydrate: 38g | Dietary Fiber: 12g | Sugars: 10g | Protein: 13g

## 63. Mushroom and Barley Soup

**Yields**: 2 servings | **Prep Time**: 15 minutes | **Cook Time**: 45 minutes

**Ingredients:**

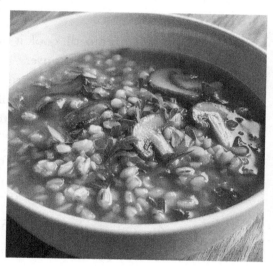

- 1 tablespoon (15ml) olive oil
- 1 small onion (about 2 ounces/60g), diced
- 2 celery stalks (about 2 ounces/60g), diced
- 2 cloves garlic, minced
- 8 ounces (225g) mixed mushrooms (like cremini and shiitake), sliced
- 1/3 cup (70g) pearl barley, rinsed
- 4 cups (960ml) low-sodium vegetable broth
- 1 bay leaf
- 1 teaspoon (2g) dried thyme
- 1/4 teaspoon (1.5g) salt
- 1/8 teaspoon (0.25g) black pepper
- 2 tablespoons (30ml) soy sauce
- 2 tablespoons (8g) fresh parsley, chopped

## INSTRUCTIONS:

1. In a large pot, heat olive oil over medium heat. Cook the onion and celery for five minutes or until they are tender. Add garlic and cook for another minute.
2. Cook the sliced mushrooms for five to seven minutes, or until they begin to brown and release their moisture.
3. Stir in barley, vegetable broth, bay leaf, thyme, salt, and pepper. Bring to a boil.
4. Reduce heat to low, cover, and simmer for about 35-40 minutes, or until barley is tender.
5. Remove bay leaf. Stir in soy sauce and taste, adjusting seasonings if needed.
6. Divide soup between two bowls and garnish with fresh parsley.

**Nutrition Per Serving:** Calories: 240 | Total Fat: 7g | Saturated Fat: 1g | Cholesterol: 0mg | Sodium: 980mg Total Carbohydrate: 38g | Dietary Fiber: 8g | Sugars: 5g | Protein: 9g

# 64. Southwest Black Bean and Corn Salad

**Yields:** 2 servings | **Prep Time:** 15 minutes | **Cook Time:** 5 minutes (for corn) | **Chill Time:** 30 minutes (optional)

**Ingredients:**

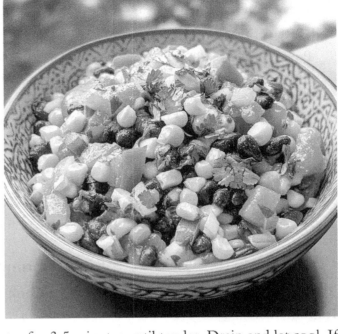

- 1 15-ounce (425g) can black beans, drained and rinsed
- 1 cup (150g) corn kernels (fresh, frozen, or canned)
- 1 medium red bell pepper (about 4 ounces/113g), diced
- 1/2 small red onion (about 2 ounces/56g), finely diced
- 1 medium tomato (about 4 ounces/113g), diced
- 1/4 cup (10g) fresh cilantro, chopped
- 1 small jalapeño pepper, seeded and minced (optional)

**For the Dressing:**

- 2 tablespoons (30ml) lime juice
- 2 tablespoons (30ml) extra virgin olive oil
- 1 teaspoon (2g) ground cumin
- 1/2 teaspoon (1g) chili powder
- 1/4 teaspoon (1.5g) salt
- 1/8 teaspoon (0.25g) black pepper

## INSTRUCTIONS:

1. If using fresh or frozen corn, cook it briefly in boiling water for 3-5 minutes until tender. Drain and let cool. If using canned corn, drain and rinse.
2. In a large bowl, mix black beans, corn, bell pepper, red onion, tomato, cilantro, and jalapeño (if using).
3. Whisk together lime juice, olive oil, chili powder, cumin, salt, and pepper in a small bowl.
4. Add the dressing to the vegetable mixture, then gently stir to blend.
5. If time allows, refrigerate the salad for 30 minutes to let the flavors meld.

**Nutrition Per Serving:** Calories: 320 | Total Fat: 14g | Saturated Fat: 2g | Cholesterol: 0mg | Sodium: 580mg Total Carbohydrate: 42g | Dietary Fiber: 13g | Sugars: 6g | Protein: 12g

# 65. Zucchini and Leek Soup

**Yields:** 2 servings | **Prep Time:** 15 minutes | **Cook Time:** 25 minutes

**Ingredients:**

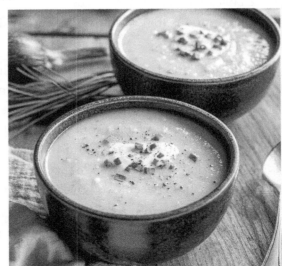

- 1 tablespoon (15ml) olive oil
- 2 medium leeks (white and light green parts only), cleaned and sliced (about 1 cup/100g)
- 2 medium zucchini (about 14 ounces/400g total), chopped
- 1 clove garlic, minced
- 3 cups (720ml) low-sodium vegetable broth
- 1/4 teaspoon (1.5g) salt
- 1/8 teaspoon (0.25g) black pepper
- 1/4 teaspoon (0.5g) dried thyme
- 2 tablespoons (30ml) heavy cream (optional)
- 2 tablespoons (8g) fresh chives, finely chopped (for garnish)

## INSTRUCTIONS:

1. Warm up the olive oil in a big pot over medium heat. Stirring occasionally, cook the leeks for 5 minutes till they become tender.
2. Stir in zucchini and garlic. Cook for another 2-3 minutes.

3. Pour in vegetable broth. Add salt, pepper, and thyme. Bring to a boil.
4. Reduce heat to low, cover, and simmer for 15-20 minutes or until zucchini is very tender.
5. Remove from heat. Use an immersion blender to puree the soup until smooth. Alternatively, carefully transfer to a blender in batches.
6. Stir in heavy cream if using. Taste and adjust seasonings if needed. Garnish with fresh chives.

**Nutrition Per Serving:** Calories: 140 | Total Fat: 8g | Saturated Fat: 2g | Cholesterol: 10mg | Sodium: 420mg
Total Carbohydrate: 16g | Dietary Fiber: 3g | Sugars: 7g | Protein: 4g

## 66. Mediterranean Couscous Salad

**Yields:** 2 servings | **Prep Time:** 15 minutes | **Cook Time:** 5 minutes | **Chill Time:** 30 minutes (optional)

**Ingredients:**

- 1/2 cup (85g) whole wheat couscous
- 3/4 cup (180ml) boiling water
- 1 tablespoon (15ml) olive oil
- 1 cup (150g) cherry tomatoes, halved
- 1/2 cucumber (about 4 ounces/113g), diced
- 1/4 red onion (about 1 ounce/28g), finely diced
- 1/4 cup (40g) pitted Kalamata olives, halved
- 1/4 cup (30g) crumbled feta cheese
- 2 tablespoons (8g) fresh parsley, chopped
- 2 tablespoons (8g) fresh mint, chopped

**For the Dressing:**

- 2 tablespoons (30ml) extra virgin olive oil
- 1 tablespoon (15ml) lemon juice
- 1 teaspoon (5g) Dijon mustard
- 1/4 teaspoon (1.5g) salt
- 1/8 teaspoon (0.25g) black pepper
- 1/4 teaspoon (0.5g) dried oregano

**INSTRUCTIONS:**

1. Place couscous in a medium bowl. Pour boiling water over it, stir, cover, and let stand for 5 minutes. Fluff with a fork and stir in 1 tablespoon olive oil. Let cool.
2. While couscous cools, prepare tomatoes, cucumber, red onion, olives, and herbs.
3. In a small bowl, whisk together olive oil, lemon juice, Dijon mustard, salt, pepper, and oregano.
4. In a large bowl, mix cooled couscous with prepared vegetables, olives, feta cheese, and herbs.
5. Pour the dressing over the salad and toss gently to combine.
6. If time allows, refrigerate the salad for 30 minutes to let the flavors meld.

**Nutrition Per Serving:** Calories: 380 | Total Fat: 24g | Saturated Fat: 5g | Cholesterol: 15mg | Sodium: 750mg
Total Carbohydrate: 35g | Dietary Fiber: 6g | Sugars: 4g | Protein: 10g

# 67. White Bean and Kale Soup

**Yields**: 2 servings | **Prep Time**: 15 minutes | **Cook Time**: 30 minutes

## Ingredients:

- 1 tablespoon (15ml) olive oil
- 1 small onion (about 2 ounces/60g), diced
- 2 cloves garlic, minced
- 1 medium carrot (about 2 ounces/60g), diced
- 1 celery stalk (about 1 ounce/30g), diced
- 1 (15-ounce/425g) can white beans (cannellini or Great Northern), drained and rinsed
- 4 cups (960ml) low-sodium vegetable broth
- 1 bay leaf
- 1/2 teaspoon (1g) dried thyme
- 1/4 teaspoon (1.5g) salt
- 1/8 teaspoon (0.25g) black pepper
- 2 cups (60g) chopped kale, stems removed
- 1 tablespoon (15ml) lemon juice
- 2 tablespoons (8g) fresh parsley, chopped

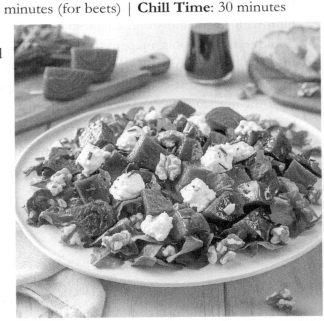

## INSTRUCTIONS:

1. In a large pot, heat olive oil over medium heat. Add onion, garlic, carrot, and celery. Simmer for 5 minutes or until the veggies begin to get tender.
2. Stir in white beans, vegetable broth, bay leaf, thyme, salt, and pepper. Bring to a boil.
3. Reduce heat to low, cover, and simmer for 15 minutes.
4. Stir in chopped kale and continue to simmer for another 5-7 minutes until kale is tender.
5. Remove bay leaf. Stir in lemon juice and taste, adjusting seasonings if needed.

**Nutrition Per Serving:** Calories: 280 | Total Fat: 7g | Saturated Fat: 1g | Cholesterol: 0mg | Sodium: 680mg
Total Carbohydrate: 42g | Dietary Fiber: 11g | Sugars: 5g | Protein: 15g

# 68. Beet and Goat Cheese Salad with Walnuts

**Yields**: 2 servings | **Prep Time**: 15 minutes | **Cook Time**: 45 minutes (for beets) | **Chill Time**: 30 minutes

## Ingredients:

- 3 medium beets (about 9 ounces/255g total), scrubbed and trimmed
- 4 cups (120g) mixed salad greens
- 2 ounces (56g) soft goat cheese, crumbled
- 1/4 cup (30g) chopped walnuts, toasted
- 2 tablespoons (8g) fresh chives, finely chopped

## For the Dressing:

- 2 tablespoons (30ml) extra virgin olive oil
- 1 tablespoon (15ml) balsamic vinegar
- 1 teaspoon (5g) Dijon mustard
- 1 teaspoon (5g) honey
- 1/4 teaspoon (1.5g) salt
- 1/8 teaspoon (0.25g) black pepper

**INSTRUCTIONS:**

1. Preheat oven to 400°F (200°C). Place the individual beets on a baking pan after wrapping them in foil. Roast for 45–60 minutes, or until tender when pierced with a fork. After letting it cool, peel and cut into wedges.
2. Mix the olive oil, honey, Dijon mustard, balsamic vinegar, salt, and pepper in a small bowl.
3. In a dry skillet, toast walnuts until fragrant and lightly golden, about 3-5 minutes. Watch carefully to prevent burning.
4. In a large bowl, toss mixed greens with half of the dressing.
5. Divide dressed greens between two plates. Top with beet wedges, crumbled goat cheese, and toasted walnuts.
6. Drizzle the remaining dressing over the salads and sprinkle with chopped chives.

**Nutrition Per Serving:** Calories: 320 | Total Fat: 25g | Saturated Fat: 6g | Cholesterol: 13mg | Sodium: 450mg
Total Carbohydrate: 18g | Dietary Fiber: 5g | Sugars: 12g | Protein: 10g

---

# 3. Flavorful Main Courses
## - Meat & Poultry
### 69. Slow Cooker Chicken and Vegetable Stew

**Yields**: 4 servings | **Prep Time**: 20 minutes | **Cook Time**: 6-8 hours on low or 3-4 hours on high

**Ingredients:**

- 1 pound (450g) boneless, skinless chicken breasts, cut into 1-inch cubes
- 2 medium carrots (about 4 ounces/113g each), peeled and chopped
- 2 celery stalks (about 2 ounces/56g each), chopped
- 1 medium onion (about 6 ounces/170g), diced
- 2 medium potatoes (about 6 ounces/170g each), peeled and cubed
- 1 cup (150g) green beans, trimmed and cut into 1-inch pieces
- 1 14-ounce (400g) can diced tomatoes
- 2 cloves garlic, minced
- 2 cups (480ml) low-sodium chicken broth
- 1 teaspoon (2g) dried thyme
- 1 teaspoon (2g) dried rosemary
- 1 bay leaf
- 1/2 teaspoon (3g) salt
- 1/4 teaspoon (0.5g) black pepper
- 2 tablespoons (16g) cornstarch (optional, for thickening)
- 1/4 cup (60ml) cold water (if using cornstarch)
- 2 tablespoons (8g) fresh parsley, chopped (for garnish)

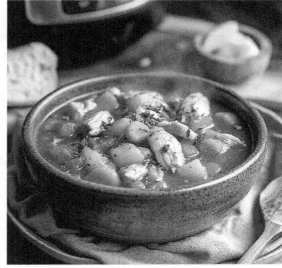

**INSTRUCTIONS:**

1. Place chicken, carrots, celery, onion, potatoes, and green beans in the slow cooker.
2. Add diced tomatoes, minced garlic, chicken broth, thyme, rosemary, bay leaf, salt, and pepper.
3. Cook, covered, for 6-8 hours on low or 3-4 hours on high, or until the chicken is thoroughly cooked and the vegetables are soft.
4. If you prefer a thicker stew, mix cornstarch with cold water in a small bowl. Stir this mixture into the stew during the last 30 minutes of cooking. Remove bay leaf before serving.

**Nutrition Per Serving:** Calories: 290 | Total Fat: 4g | Saturated Fat: 1g | Cholesterol: 65mg | Sodium: 520mg
Total Carbohydrate: 34g | Dietary Fiber: 6g | Sugars: 7g | Protein: 29g

## 70. Turkey Meatloaf with Oats

**Yields**: 4 servings | **Prep Time**: 15 minutes | **Cook Time**: 45-50 minutes

**Ingredients:**

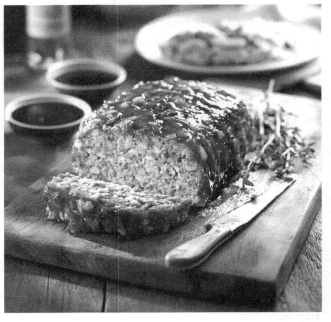

- 1 pound (450g) lean ground turkey
- 3/4 cup (60g) old-fashioned rolled oats
- 1 small onion (about 4 ounces/113g), finely diced
- 1 medium carrot (about 2 ounces/56g), grated
- 1 large egg, lightly beaten
- 1/4 cup (60ml) unsweetened almond milk (or regular milk)
- 2 tablespoons (30g) tomato paste
- 1 teaspoon (3g) garlic powder
- 1 teaspoon (2g) dried thyme
- 1 teaspoon (6g) salt
- 1/4 teaspoon (0.5g) black pepper

**For the Glaze:**

- 2 tablespoons (30g) tomato paste
- 1 tablespoon (15ml) balsamic vinegar
- 1 teaspoon (5g) honey

### INSTRUCTIONS:

1. Set oven to 375°F (190°C).
2. In a large bowl, mix ground turkey, oats, onion, carrot, egg, almond milk, tomato paste, garlic powder, thyme, salt, and pepper. Mix well, but don't overmix.
3. The ingredients can be shaped into a loaf on a baking sheet covered with parchment paper or transferred to a 9 by 5-inch loaf pan.
4. In a small bowl, mix tomato paste, balsamic vinegar, and honey.
5. Spread the glaze evenly over the top of the meatloaf.
6. Cook for 45 to 50 minutes, or until 165°F (74°C) is reached internally.

**Nutrition Per Serving:** Calories: 270 | Total Fat: 11g | Saturated Fat: 3g | Cholesterol: 115mg | Sodium: 680mg
Total Carbohydrate: 18g | Dietary Fiber: 3g | Sugars: 5g | Protein: 28g

## 71. Grilled Pork Tenderloin with Apple Chutney

**Yields**: 4 servings | **Prep Time**: 20 minutes (plus 1 hour marinating time) | **Cook Time**: 20 minutes

**Ingredients:**

**For the Pork:**

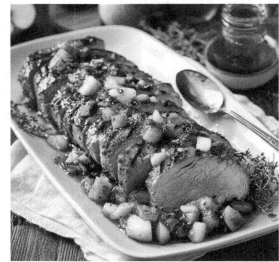

- 1 pound (450g) pork tenderloin
- 2 tablespoons (30ml) olive oil
- 2 cloves garlic, minced
- 1 teaspoon (2g) dried thyme
- 1 teaspoon (6g) salt
- 1/4 teaspoon (0.5g) black pepper

**For the Apple Chutney:**

- 2 medium apples (about 7 ounces/200g each), peeled, cored, and diced
- 1/4 cup (40g) finely chopped red onion

- 2 tablespoons (30ml) apple cider vinegar
- 2 tablespoons (30g) honey
- 1/4 teaspoon (0.5g) ground cinnamon
- 1/8 teaspoon (0.25g) ground ginger
- Pinch of salt

## INSTRUCTIONS:

1. Mix olive oil, thyme, garlic, salt, and pepper in a small bowl. Apply this mixture evenly over the tenderloin of pork. Cover and refrigerate for 1 hour.
2. Preheat the grill to medium-high heat.
3. While the grill is heating, combine all chutney ingredients in a small saucepan. Over medium heat, bring to a simmer, then lower heat to low and cook, stirring periodically, until the mixture thickens and the apples become mushy, about 15 minutes. Set aside.
4. Grill the pork tenderloin for 15-20 minutes, turning every 5 minutes, until the internal temperature reaches 145°F (63°C).

**Nutrition Per Serving:** Calories: 270 | Total Fat: 10g | Saturated Fat: 2g | Cholesterol: 75mg | Sodium: 650mg Total Carbohydrate: 20g | Dietary Fiber: 2g | Sugars: 17g | Protein: 26g

## 72. Beef and Broccoli Stir-Fry with Brown Rice

**Yields**: 4 servings | **Prep Time**: 20 minutes | **Cook Time**: 20 minutes

### Ingredients:

### For the Stir-Fry:

- 1 pound (450g) lean beef sirloin, sliced thinly against the grain
- 4 cups (280g) broccoli florets
- 1 medium red bell pepper (about 6 ounces/170g), sliced
- 2 cloves garlic, minced
- 1 tablespoon (15ml) grated fresh ginger
- 2 tablespoons (30ml) vegetable oil
- 2 cups (370g) cooked brown rice

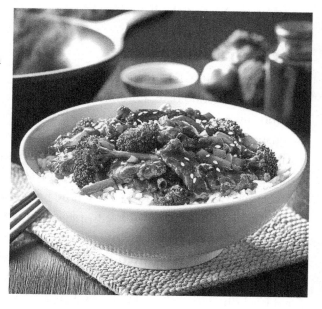

### For the Sauce:

- 1/4 cup (60ml) low-sodium soy sauce
- 1/4 cup (60ml) low-sodium beef broth
- 2 tablespoons (30ml) oyster sauce
- 1 tablespoon (15g) cornstarch
- 1 teaspoon (5g) honey

## INSTRUCTIONS:

1. In a small bowl, whisk together soy sauce, beef broth, oyster sauce, cornstarch, and honey. Set aside.
2. If not prepared, cook brown rice according to package instructions.
3. Heat 1 tablespoon oil in a large wok or skillet over high heat. Add beef and stir-fry for 2-3 minutes until browned. Remove from wok and set aside.
4. In the same wok, add the remaining oil. Stir-fry broccoli and bell pepper for 3-4 minutes until crisp-tender.
5. Add garlic and ginger to the wok and stir-fry for 30 seconds. Return beef to the wok.
6. Pour the sauce over the beef and vegetables. Cook, stirring constantly, until the sauce thickens and coats everything evenly, about 2-3 minutes.

**Nutrition Per Serving:** Calories: 420 | Total Fat: 15g | Saturated Fat: 4g | Cholesterol: 70mg | Sodium: 650mg Total Carbohydrate: 40g | Dietary Fiber: 5g | Sugars: 5g | Protein: 32g

# 73. Baked Chicken Fajitas

**Yields**: 4 servings | **Prep Time**: 15 minutes | **Cook Time**: 25-30 minutes

**Ingredients:**

- 1 pound (450g) boneless, skinless chicken breasts, sliced into strips
- 1 red bell pepper, sliced
- 1 yellow bell pepper, sliced
- 1 green bell pepper, sliced
- 1 medium onion, sliced
- 2 tablespoons (30ml) olive oil
- 2 cloves garlic, minced
- 1 teaspoon (2g) ground cumin
- 1 teaspoon (2g) chili powder
- 1/2 teaspoon (1g) smoked paprika
- 1/2 teaspoon (3g) salt
- 1/4 teaspoon (0.5g) black pepper
- Juice of 1 lime
- 8 small whole wheat tortillas (6-inch diameter)

**Optional Toppings:**

- 1/2 cup (120g) plain Greek yogurt
- 1/4 cup (10g) fresh cilantro, chopped
- 1 avocado, sliced

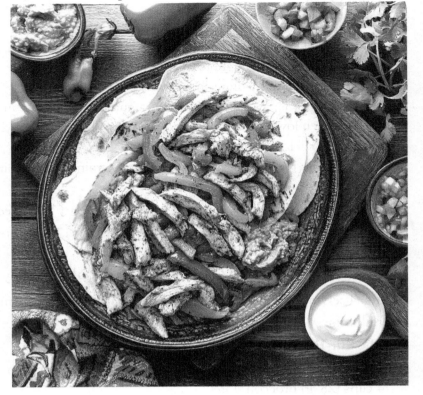

## INSTRUCTIONS:

1. Set oven to 400°F (200°C).
2. In a large baking dish, combine chicken strips, bell peppers, and onion.
3. Add olive oil, cumin, smoked paprika, chili powder, minced garlic, and salt & pepper to a small bowl. Toss to ensure even coating after pouring this mixture over the chicken and veggies.
4. Place the baking dish in the preheated oven and bake for 25-30 minutes, stirring once halfway through, until the chicken is cooked through and the vegetables are tender.
5. Remove from oven and squeeze lime juice over the fajita mixture.
6. Warm the tortillas according to package instructions. Serve the fajita mixture with warm tortillas and optional toppings.

**Nutrition Per Serving (including 2 tortillas, without optional toppings):**

Calories: 380 | Total Fat: 12g | Saturated Fat: 2g | Cholesterol: 65mg | Sodium: 580mg
Total Carbohydrate: 40g | Dietary Fiber: 6g | Sugars: 5g | Protein: 30g

# 74. Turkey and Spinach Stuffed Bell Peppers

**Yields**: 4 servings | **Prep Time**: 20 minutes | **Cook Time**: 35-40 minutes

**Ingredients:**

- 4 large bell peppers (any color), halved lengthwise and seeds removed
- 1 pound (450g) lean ground turkey
- 1 cup (180g) cooked brown rice
- 2 cups (60g) fresh spinach, chopped
- 1 small onion (about 4 ounces/113g), finely diced
- 2 cloves garlic, minced
- 1 14-ounce (400g) can diced tomatoes, drained

- 1 teaspoon (2g) dried oregano
- 1 teaspoon (2g) ground cumin
- 1/2 teaspoon (3g) salt
- 1/4 teaspoon (0.5g) black pepper
- 1/2 cup (56g) shredded low-fat mozzarella cheese
- 2 tablespoons (8g) fresh parsley, chopped (for garnish)

## INSTRUCTIONS:

1. Set oven to 375°F (190°C).
2. Place halved peppers in a large baking dish.
3. In a large skillet over medium heat, cook ground turkey until no longer pink, breaking it up with a spoon as it cooks.
4. Add onion and garlic to the skillet and cook for another 2-3 minutes until onion is softened.
5. Stir in cooked rice, chopped spinach, diced tomatoes, oregano, cumin, salt, and pepper. Cook until spinach is wilted, about 2 minutes.
6. Spoon the turkey mixture into the bell pepper halves.
7. Cover the baking dish with foil and bake for 30-35 minutes, until peppers are tender.
8. Uncover, sprinkle with mozzarella cheese, and bake for 5 minutes until cheese is melted.

**Nutrition Per Serving (2 pepper halves):** Calories: 340 | Total Fat: 12g | Saturated Fat: 3g | Cholesterol: 70mg Sodium: 520mg | Total Carbohydrate: 30g | Dietary Fiber: 6g | Sugars: 8g | Protein: 32g

## 75. Grilled Lemon Herb Chicken

**Yields:** 4 servings | **Prep Time:** 10 minutes (plus 30 minutes to 2 hours marinating time)
**Cook Time:** 12-15 minutes

### Ingredients:

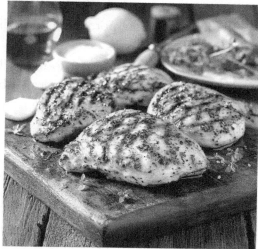

- 4 boneless, skinless chicken breasts (about 6 ounces/170g each)
- 1/4 cup (60ml) olive oil
- Zest and juice of 2 lemons
- 3 cloves garlic, minced
- 2 tablespoons (8g) fresh oregano, chopped (or 2 teaspoons dried)
- 2 tablespoons (8g) fresh thyme, chopped (or 2 teaspoons dried)
- 1 teaspoon (6g) salt
- 1/4 teaspoon (0.5g) black pepper
- Lemon wedges for serving

## INSTRUCTIONS:

1. In a bowl, whisk together olive oil, lemon zest, lemon juice, minced garlic, oregano, thyme, salt, and pepper.
2. Place chicken breasts in a large zip-top bag or shallow dish. Make sure the chicken is evenly coated after pouring the marinade over it. Refrigerate for at least 30 minutes and up to two hours after sealing or covering.
3. Set grill to medium-high heat.
4. Remove chicken from marinade, letting excess drip off. The interior temperature should reach 165°F (74°C) after grilling for 6–7 minutes on each side.

**Nutrition Per Serving:** Calories: 280 | Total Fat: 15g | Saturated Fat: 2g | Cholesterol: 85mg | Sodium: 650mg Total Carbohydrate: 2g | Dietary Fiber: 1g | Sugars: 0g | Protein: 34g

# 76. Beef and Barley Casserole

**Yields**: 6 servings | **Prep Time**: 20 minutes | **Cook Time**: 1 hour 30 minutes

**Ingredients:**

- 1 pound (450g) lean beef stew meat, cut into 1-inch cubes
- 1 cup (200g) pearl barley, rinsed
- 1 medium onion, diced
- 2 medium carrots, diced
- 2 celery stalks, diced
- 2 cloves garlic, minced
- 1 14-ounce (400g) can diced tomatoes
- 4 cups (960ml) low-sodium beef broth
- 1 tablespoon (15ml) olive oil
- 1 teaspoon (2g) dried thyme
- 1 teaspoon (2g) dried rosemary
- 2 bay leaves
- 1 teaspoon (6g) salt
- 1/4 teaspoon (0.5g) black pepper
- 2 tablespoons (8g) fresh parsley, chopped (for garnish)

## INSTRUCTIONS:

1. Set oven to 350°F (175°C).
2. Heat olive oil over medium-high heat in a large oven-safe Dutch oven or casserole dish. Add beef cubes and brown on all sides for about 5 minutes. Remove beef and set aside.
3. In the same pot, add onion, carrots, and celery. Cook for 5 minutes until vegetables start to soften. Add garlic and cook for another minute.
4. Return beef to the pot. Add barley, diced tomatoes, beef broth, thyme, rosemary, bay leaves, salt, and pepper. Stir to combine.
5. Cover the pot and transfer to the preheated oven. Bake for 1 hour and 30 minutes, or until beef is tender and barley is cooked. Remove bay leaves before serving. Ladle into bowls and garnish with fresh parsley.

**Nutrition Per Serving:** Calories: 320 | Total Fat: 9g | Saturated Fat: 3g | Cholesterol: 50mg | Sodium: 580mg
Total Carbohydrate: 38g | Dietary Fiber: 8g | Sugars: 4g | Protein: 25g

---

## - Fish & Seafood

## 77. Baked Salmon with Dill Sauce

**Yields**: 4 servings | **Prep Time**: 10 minutes | **Cook Time**: 15-18 minutes

**Ingredients:**

**For the Salmon:**

- 4 salmon fillets (about 6 ounces/170g each)
- 1 tablespoon (15ml) olive oil
- 1/2 teaspoon (3g) salt
- 1/4 teaspoon (0.5g) black pepper
- 1 lemon, sliced

**For the Dill Sauce:**

- 1/2 cup (120g) plain Greek yogurt
- 2 tablespoons (8g) fresh dill, finely chopped

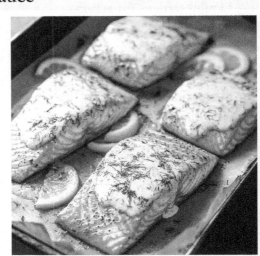

- 1 tablespoon (15ml) lemon juice
- 1 clove garlic, minced
- 1/4 teaspoon (1.5g) salt
- 1/8 teaspoon (0.25g) black pepper

## INSTRUCTIONS:

1. Set oven to 400°F (200°C).
2. Place salmon fillets on a baking sheet lined with parchment paper. Brush with olive oil and season with salt and pepper.
3. Place lemon slices on top of and around the salmon fillets.
4. Cook in the preheated oven for 15-18 minutes or until salmon flakes easily with a fork.
5. While salmon is baking, mix Greek yogurt, chopped dill, lemon juice, minced garlic, salt, and pepper in a small bowl. Plate the baked salmon and serve with a dollop of dill sauce on the side.

**Nutrition Per Serving:** Calories: 300 | Total Fat: 18g | Saturated Fat: 3g | Cholesterol: 80mg | Sodium: 450mg Total Carbohydrate: 3g | Dietary Fiber: 0g | Sugars: 2g | Protein: 32g

## 78. Shrimp and Vegetable Skewers

**Yields**: 4 servings | **Prep Time**: 20 minutes (plus 30 minutes marinating time) | **Cook Time**: 8-10 minutes

### Ingredients:

**For the Skewers:**

- 1 pound (450g) large shrimp, peeled and deveined
- 1 zucchini, cut into 1-inch chunks
- 1 yellow bell pepper, cut into 1-inch pieces
- 1 red onion, cut into 1-inch pieces
- 1 pint of cherry tomatoes

**For the Marinade:**

- 1/4 cup (60ml) olive oil
- 2 tablespoons (30ml) lemon juice
- 2 cloves garlic, minced
- 1 teaspoon (2g) dried oregano
- 1/2 teaspoon (3g) salt
- 1/4 teaspoon (0.5g) black pepper

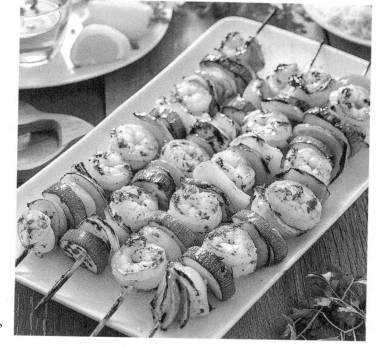

### INSTRUCTIONS:

1. In a bowl, whisk together olive oil, lemon juice, minced garlic, oregano, salt, and pepper.
2. Place shrimp in a large zip-top bag and add half of the marinade. Seal and refrigerate for 30 minutes.
3. In another large bowl, toss the zucchini, bell pepper, red onion, and cherry tomatoes with the remaining marinade.
4. Set grill to medium-high heat.
5. Thread the marinated shrimp and vegetables onto skewers, alternating ingredients.
6. Cook skewers on the preheated grill for 2-3 minutes per side, or until shrimp are pink and opaque and vegetables are slightly charred.

**Nutrition Per Serving (2 skewers):** Calories: 240 | Total Fat: 14g | Saturated Fat: 2g | Cholesterol: 170mg Sodium: 450mg | Total Carbohydrate: 10g | Dietary Fiber: 2g | Sugars: 5g | Protein: 22g

# 79. Tuna Nicoise Salad

**Yields:** 4 servings | **Prep Time:** 20 minutes | **Cook Time:** 15 minutes (for eggs and potatoes)

**Ingredients:**

- 2 6-ounce (170g) cans of chunk light tuna in water, drained
- 4 cups (120g) mixed salad greens
- 1/2 pound (225g) small new potatoes, boiled and quartered
- 1/2 pound (225g) green beans, trimmed and blanched
- 4 hard-boiled eggs, peeled and quartered
- 1 cup (150g) cherry tomatoes, halved
- 1/2 cup (60g) pitted Kalamata olives
- 1/4 red onion, thinly sliced

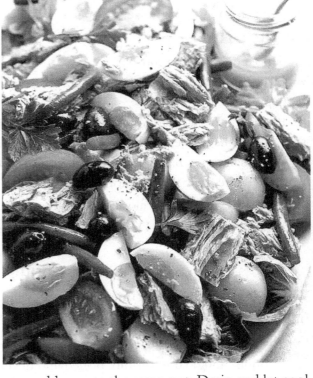

**For the Dressing:**

- 1/4 cup (60ml) extra virgin olive oil
- 2 tablespoons (30ml) red wine vinegar
- 1 tablespoon (15g) Dijon mustard
- 1 clove garlic, minced
- 1/2 teaspoon (3g) salt
- 1/4 teaspoon (0.5g) black pepper
- 1 tablespoon (4g) fresh thyme leaves (or 1 teaspoon dried)

**INSTRUCTIONS:**

1. Boil potatoes until tender, about 15 minutes. In the last 7 minutes, add eggs to the same pot. Drain and let cool.
2. In a separate pot of boiling water, cook green beans for 3-4 minutes until crisp-tender. Drain and rinse with cold water.
3. Mix the olive oil, red wine vinegar, Dijon mustard, minced garlic, salt, pepper, and thyme in a small bowl.
4. Arrange mixed greens in a large bowl or on individual plates. Top with tuna, quartered potatoes, green beans, quartered eggs, cherry tomatoes, olives, and red onion slices.
5. Drizzle the prepared dressing over the salad just before serving.

**Nutrition Per Serving:** Calories: 380 | Total Fat: 22g | Saturated Fat: 4g | Cholesterol: 225mg | Sodium: 650mg
Total Carbohydrate: 24g | Dietary Fiber: 5g | Sugars: 4g | Protein: 25g

# 80. Grilled Trout with Lemon and Herbs

**Yields:** 4 servings | **Prep Time:** 15 minutes | **Cook Time:** 10-12 minutes

**Ingredients:**

- 4 whole trout (about 12 ounces/340g each), cleaned and gutted
- 2 tablespoons (30ml) olive oil
- 2 lemons, 1 sliced and 1 for juicing
- 4 sprigs fresh rosemary
- 4 sprigs fresh thyme
- 4 cloves garlic, thinly sliced
- 1 teaspoon (6g) salt
- 1/2 teaspoon (1g) black pepper
- 1/4 cup (10g) fresh parsley, chopped (for garnish)

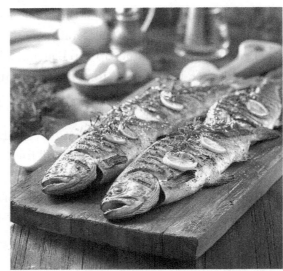

## INSTRUCTIONS:

1. Preheat the grill to medium-high heat.
2. Rinse trout and pat dry with paper towels. Rub each fish inside and out with olive oil. Season inside and out with salt and pepper.
3. Place 2-3 lemon slices, 1 sprig each of rosemary and thyme, and a few garlic slices inside each trout cavity.
4. Place trout on the preheated grill. Cook for 5-6 minutes per side or until the skin is crispy and the flesh flakes easily with a fork.
5. Squeeze juice from the remaining lemon over the grilled fish.
6. Transfer trout to plates, garnish with chopped parsley, and serve immediately.

**Nutrition Per Serving:** Calories: 300 | Total Fat: 16g | Saturated Fat: 3g | Cholesterol: 85mg | Sodium: 650mg Total Carbohydrate: 2g | Dietary Fiber: 1g | Sugars: 0g | Protein: 35g

## 81. Cod Fish Tacos with Cabbage Slaw

**Yields:** 4 servings (2 tacos per serving) | **Prep Time:** 20 minutes | **Cook Time:** 10 minutes

### Ingredients:

**For the Fish:**

- 1 pound (450g) cod fillets
- 1 tablespoon (15ml) olive oil
- 1 teaspoon (2g) ground cumin
- 1 teaspoon (2g) chili powder
- 1/2 teaspoon (3g) salt
- 1/4 teaspoon (0.5g) black pepper

**For the Cabbage Slaw:**

- 2 cups (140g) shredded green cabbage
- 1/2 cup (50g) shredded carrots
- 1/4 cup (10g) chopped cilantro
- 2 tablespoons (30ml) lime juice
- 1 tablespoon (15ml) olive oil
- 1/4 teaspoon (1.5g) salt

**For Assembly:**

- 8 small corn tortillas (6-inch diameter)
- 1 avocado, sliced
- Lime wedges for serving

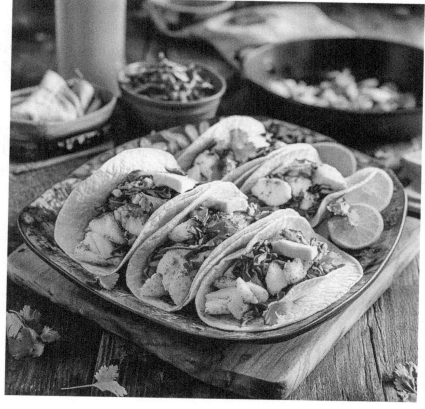

### INSTRUCTIONS:

1. In a medium bowl, combine cabbage, carrots, cilantro, lime juice, olive oil, and salt. Toss well and set aside to let flavors meld.
2. In a small bowl, mix cumin, chili powder, salt, and pepper. Rub this mixture over the cod fillets.
3. Heat olive oil in a large skillet over medium-high heat. Add cod and cook for 3-4 minutes per side or until fish flakes easily with a fork.
4. Heat corn tortillas according to package instructions or in a dry skillet for about 30 seconds per side.
5. Flake the cooked cod into large pieces. Fill each tortilla with fish, then top with cabbage slaw and sliced avocado.

**Nutrition Per Serving (2 tacos):** Calories: 320 | Total Fat: 15g | Saturated Fat: 2g | Cholesterol: 50mg Sodium: 520mg | Total Carbohydrate: 28g | Dietary Fiber: 7g | Sugars: 3g | Protein: 22g

# 82. Baked Tilapia with Tomato and Olive Topping

**Yields:** 4 servings | **Prep Time:** 15 minutes **Cook Time:** 15-20 minutes

**Ingredients:**

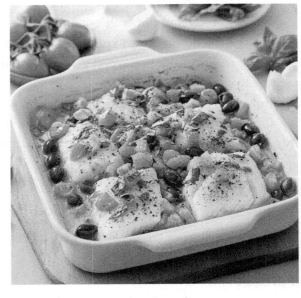

- 4 tilapia fillets (about 6 ounces/170g each)
- 2 tablespoons (30ml) olive oil, divided
- 1/2 teaspoon (3g) salt
- 1/4 teaspoon (0.5g) black pepper
- 2 medium tomatoes, diced
- 1/4 cup (35g) pitted Kalamata olives, chopped
- 2 cloves garlic, minced
- 1 tablespoon (4g) fresh basil, chopped
- 1 tablespoon (15ml) lemon juice
- 1/4 teaspoon (0.5g) dried oregano
- Lemon wedges for serving

**INSTRUCTIONS:**

1. Set oven to 400°F (200°C).
2. Place tilapia fillets in a baking dish. Brush with 1 tablespoon olive oil and season with salt and pepper.
3. In a bowl, combine diced tomatoes, chopped olives, minced garlic, chopped basil, lemon juice, oregano, and the remaining 1 tablespoon olive oil. Mix well.
4. Spoon the tomato and olive mixture over the tilapia fillets.
5. The fish should flake readily with a fork after 15 to 20 minutes of baking the baking dish in the preheated oven.

**Nutrition Per Serving:** Calories: 240 | Total Fat: 11g | Saturated Fat: 2g | Cholesterol: 85mg | Sodium: 450mg

Total Carbohydrate: 4g | Dietary Fiber: 1g | Sugars: 2g | Protein: 32g

## 83. Lentil and Mushroom Loaf

**Yields:** 6 servings | **Prep Time:** 20 minutes | **Cook Time:** 50 minutes

**Ingredients:**

- 1 cup (200g) green or brown lentils, rinsed
- 2 1/2 cups (600ml) vegetable broth
- 1 tablespoon (15ml) olive oil
- 1 medium onion, finely chopped
- 2 celery stalks, finely chopped
- 2 medium carrots, finely chopped
- 8 ounces (225g) mushrooms, finely chopped
- 3 cloves garlic, minced
- 1 cup (90g) old-fashioned rolled oats
- 1/4 cup (60ml) tomato paste
- 2 tablespoons (30ml) soy sauce or tamari
- 1 tablespoon (7g) ground flaxseed
- 1 teaspoon (2g) dried thyme
- 1 teaspoon (2g) dried oregano
- 1/2 teaspoon (3g) salt
- 1/4 teaspoon (0.5g) black pepper

**For the Glaze:**

- 2 tablespoons (30ml) tomato paste
- 1 tablespoon (15ml) balsamic vinegar
- 1 tablespoon (15ml) maple syrup

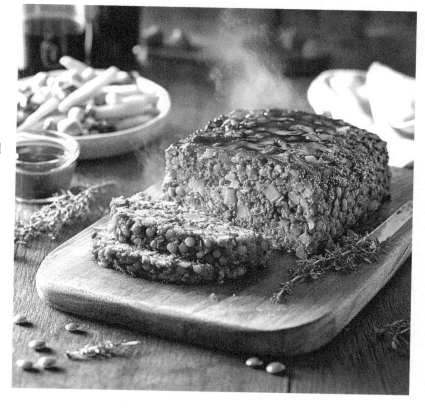

## INSTRUCTIONS:

1. Combine lentils and vegetable broth in a medium saucepan. Bring to a boil, then reduce heat and simmer for about 20 minutes or until lentils are tender. Drain any excess liquid.
2. Set oven to 375°F (190°C).
3. Heat olive oil over medium heat in a large skillet. Add onion, celery, and carrots. Cook for 5-7 minutes until softened. Add mushrooms and garlic, cooking for another 5 minutes.
4. In a large bowl, mix cooked lentils, sautéed vegetables, oats, tomato paste, soy sauce, ground flaxseed, thyme, oregano, salt, and pepper.
5. Press the mixture into a 9x5-inch loaf pan lined with parchment paper.
6. In a small bowl, mix tomato paste, balsamic vinegar, and maple syrup. Spread over the top of the loaf.
7. Place in preheated oven and bake for 30-35 minutes, until firm and golden on top.

**Nutrition Per Serving:** Calories: 220 | Total Fat: 4g | Saturated Fat: 0.5g | Cholesterol: 0mg | Sodium: 480mg
Total Carbohydrate: 38g | Dietary Fiber: 11g | Sugars: 7g | Protein: 12g

## 84. Stuffed Portobello Mushrooms

**Yields:** 4 servings | **Prep Time:** 20 minutes | **Cook Time:** 25 minutes

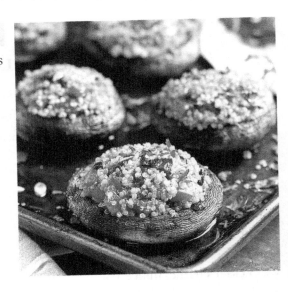

**Ingredients:**

- 4 large portobello mushrooms
- 1 cup (185g) cooked quinoa
- 1 tablespoon (15ml) olive oil
- 1 small onion, finely chopped
- 1 red bell pepper, diced
- 2 cloves garlic, minced
- 1 cup (30g) baby spinach, roughly chopped
- 1/4 cup (40g) sun-dried tomatoes, chopped
- 2 tablespoons (8g) nutritional yeast
- 1 tablespoon (15ml) balsamic vinegar
- 1 teaspoon (2g) dried oregano
- 1/2 teaspoon (3g) salt
- 1/4 teaspoon (0.5g) black pepper
- 1/4 cup (30g) pine nuts (optional)

### INSTRUCTIONS:

1. Set oven to 375°F (190°C).
2. Clean portobello mushrooms and remove stems. Chop stems finely and set aside.
3. Heat olive oil in a large skillet over medium heat. Add onion and bell pepper, cooking for 5 minutes until softened. Add garlic and chopped mushroom stems, cooking for another 2 minutes.
4. In a large bowl, combine cooked quinoa, sautéed vegetables, spinach, sun-dried tomatoes, nutritional yeast, balsamic vinegar, oregano, salt, and pepper. Mix well.
5. Place mushroom caps on a baking sheet, gill side up. Fill each mushroom generously with the quinoa mixture.
6. Place in preheated oven and bake for 20-25 minutes, until mushrooms are tender and filling is heated through.
7. If using pine nuts, sprinkle them over the stuffed mushrooms in the last 5 minutes of baking.

**Nutrition Per Serving (1 stuffed mushroom):** Calories: 220 | Total Fat: 9g | Saturated Fat: 1g | Cholesterol: 0mg
Sodium: 320mg | Total Carbohydrate: 30g | Dietary Fiber: 5g | Sugars: 6g | Protein: 9g

## 85. Chickpea and Spinach Curry

**Yields:** 4 servings | **Prep Time:** 15 minutes
**Cook Time:** 25 minutes

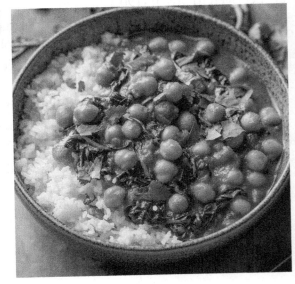

**Ingredients:**

- 2 15-ounce (425g) cans chickpeas, drained and rinsed
- 1 tablespoon (15ml) coconut oil
- 1 large onion, finely chopped
- 3 cloves garlic, minced
- 1 tablespoon (15g) grated fresh ginger
- 2 teaspoons (4g) ground cumin
- 2 teaspoons (4g) ground coriander
- 1 teaspoon (2g) turmeric
- 1/4 teaspoon (0.5g) cayenne pepper (optional)
- 1 14-ounce (400ml) can diced tomatoes
- 1 14-ounce (400ml) can coconut milk
- 4 cups (120g) fresh spinach, roughly chopped
- Salt to taste
- Juice of 1 lemon
- 1/4 cup (10g) fresh cilantro, chopped

**For Serving:**

- Cooked brown rice or quinoa

## INSTRUCTIONS:

1. Heat coconut oil in a large pot over medium heat. Add onion and cook for 5 minutes until softened. Add garlic and ginger, cooking for another minute.
2. Stir in cumin, coriander, turmeric, and cayenne (if using). Cook for 1 minute until fragrant.
3. Add chickpeas, diced tomatoes, and coconut milk. Bring to a simmer and cook for 15 minutes, stirring occasionally.
4. Stir in chopped spinach and cook for 2-3 minutes until wilted. Add salt to taste and stir in lemon juice.
5. Remove from heat and stir in fresh cilantro. Spoon curry over cooked brown rice or quinoa.

**Nutrition Per Serving (without rice):** Calories: 380 | Total Fat: 22g | Saturated Fat: 16g | Cholesterol: 0mg Sodium: 390mg | Total Carbohydrate: 38g | Dietary Fiber: 11g | Sugars: 8g | Protein: 12g

## 86. Quinoa-Stuffed Acorn Squash

**Yields:** 4 servings | **Prep Time:** 20 minutes | **Cook Time:** 40-45 minutes

### Ingredients:

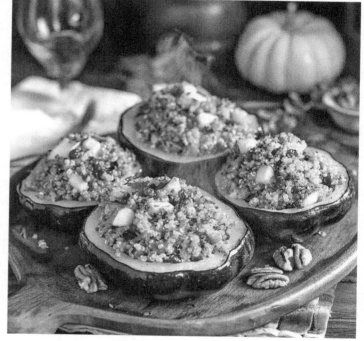

- 2 medium acorn squash, halved and seeds removed
- 2 tablespoons (30ml) olive oil, divided
- 1 cup (185g) quinoa, rinsed
- 2 cups (480ml) vegetable broth
- 1 small onion, finely chopped
- 2 cloves garlic, minced
- 1 medium apple, diced
- 1/4 cup (40g) dried cranberries
- 1/4 cup (30g) pecans, chopped
- 1 teaspoon (2g) ground cinnamon
- 1/2 teaspoon (1g) dried thyme
- 1/4 teaspoon (0.5g) ground nutmeg
- Salt and pepper to taste
- 2 tablespoons (8g) fresh parsley, chopped

## INSTRUCTIONS:

1. Set oven to 400°F (200°C).
2. Brush the cut sides of acorn squash with 1 tablespoon olive oil. Place cut-side down on a baking sheet and roast for 30-35 minutes, until tender.
3. Combine quinoa and vegetable broth in a medium saucepan. After 15 to 20 minutes of simmering covered over a reduced heat, the quinoa should be frothy.
4. Heat remaining olive oil over medium heat in a large skillet. Add onion and garlic, cooking until softened, about 5 minutes. Add diced apple and cook for another 3 minutes.
5. In a large bowl, mix cooked quinoa, sautéed onion and apple mixture, dried cranberries, chopped pecans, cinnamon, thyme, and nutmeg. Season with salt and pepper to taste.
6. Once the squash halves are tender, flip them over and fill each with the quinoa mixture.
7. Return stuffed squash to the oven for 5-10 minutes to heat through. Garnish with fresh parsley before serving.

**Nutrition Per Serving (1/2 stuffed squash):** Calories: 340 | Total Fat: 14g | Saturated Fat: 2g | Cholesterol: 0mg Sodium: 280mg | Total Carbohydrate: 52g | Dietary Fiber: 7g | Sugars: 11g | Protein: 8g

# 87. Vegetable and Tofu Stir-Fry

**Yields:** 4 servings | **Prep Time:** 20 minutes | **Cook Time:** 15 minutes

## Ingredients:

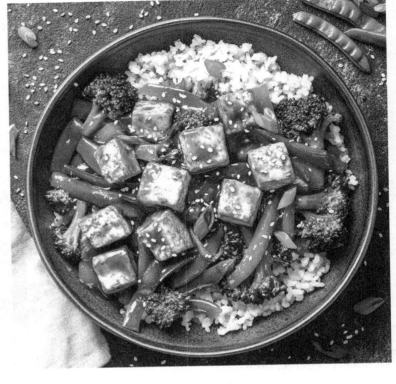

- 14 ounces (400g) extra-firm tofu, pressed and cut into 1-inch cubes
- 2 tablespoons (30g) cornstarch
- 3 tablespoons (45ml) vegetable oil, divided
- 1 medium onion, sliced
- 2 cloves garlic, minced
- 1 tablespoon (15g) grated fresh ginger
- 1 red bell pepper, sliced
- 2 cups (140g) broccoli florets
- 1 cup (100g) snap peas
- 1 cup (70g) sliced carrots
- 1/4 cup (60ml) low-sodium soy sauce or tamari
- 2 tablespoons (30ml) rice vinegar
- 1 tablespoon (15ml) maple syrup
- 1/4 cup (60ml) vegetable broth
- 1 teaspoon (5g) sesame oil
- 2 green onions, sliced (for garnish)
- 1 tablespoon (9g) sesame seeds (for garnish)

## For Serving:

- Cooked brown rice or cauliflower rice

## INSTRUCTIONS:

1. Toss tofu cubes with cornstarch to coat evenly.
2. Heat 2 tablespoons oil in a large wok or skillet over medium-high heat. Add tofu and cook for 5-7 minutes, turning occasionally, until golden on all sides. Remove and set aside.
3. Add the remaining 1 tablespoon oil to the same wok. Add onion, garlic, and ginger, stir-frying for 1 minute. Add bell pepper, broccoli, snap peas, and carrots. Stir-fry for 4-5 minutes until vegetables are crisp-tender.
4. In a small bowl, whisk together soy sauce, rice vinegar, maple syrup, and vegetable broth.
5. Add cooked tofu back to the wok with the vegetables. Pour sauce over and toss to coat everything evenly. Cook for another 2-3 minutes until heated through.
6. Remove from heat and stir in sesame oil.
7. Divide stir-fry among plates and serve over brown rice or cauliflower rice. Garnish with sliced green onions and sesame seeds.

**Nutrition Per Serving (without rice):** Calories: 260 | Total Fat: 16g | Saturated Fat: 2g | Cholesterol: 0mg Sodium: 580mg | Total Carbohydrate: 20g | Dietary Fiber: 5g | Sugars: 10g | Protein: 14g

# 88. Black Bean and Sweet Potato Tacos

**Yields:** 4 servings (2 tacos per serving) | **Prep Time:** 15 minutes | **Cook Time:** 25 minutes

## Ingredients:

- 2 medium sweet potatoes (about 1 pound/450g), peeled and diced
- 1 tablespoon (15ml) olive oil
- 1 teaspoon (2g) ground cumin
- 1 teaspoon (2g) chili powder
- 1/2 teaspoon (3g) salt
- 1 15-ounce (425g) can black beans, drained and rinsed
- 1 small red onion, finely diced
- 1 lime, juiced
- 8 small corn tortillas
- 2 cups (60g) shredded lettuce or cabbage
- 1 avocado, sliced
- 1/4 cup (10g) fresh cilantro, chopped

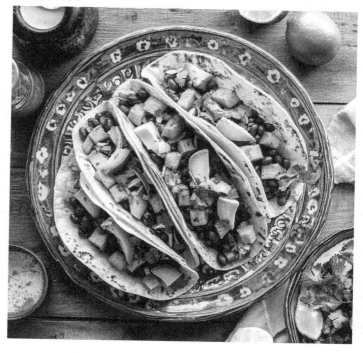

### For the Cashew Cream (optional):

- 1 cup (150g) raw cashews, soaked for at least 2 hours
- 1/4 cup (60ml) water
- 2 tablespoons (30ml) lime juice
- 1/4 teaspoon (1.5g) salt

## INSTRUCTIONS:

1. Preheat oven to 400°F (200°C). Toss diced sweet potatoes with olive oil, cumin, chili powder, and salt. Spread on a baking sheet and roast for 20-25 minutes, stirring halfway through, until tender.
2. Warm the black beans in a small pot over medium heat.
3. Drain soaked cashews and blend with water, lime juice, and salt until smooth.
4. Mix diced red onion with lime juice and set aside.
5. Heat corn tortillas according to package instructions.
6. Fill each tortilla with roasted sweet potatoes, black beans, lettuce or cabbage, avocado slices, lime-marinated red onion, and fresh cilantro.
7. Drizzle with cashew cream if using, and serve immediately.

**Nutrition Per Serving (2 tacos, without cashew cream):** Calories: 380 | Total Fat: 11g | Saturated Fat: 2g Cholesterol: 0mg | Sodium: 520mg | Total Carbohydrate: 62g | Dietary Fiber: 15g | Sugars: 7g | Protein: 12g

## 4. Deliciously Gut-Friendly Sides

## 89. Roasted Brussels Sprouts with Balsamic Glaze

**Yields**: 4 servings | **Prep Time**: 10 minutes | **Cook Time**: 20-25 minutes

**Ingredients:**

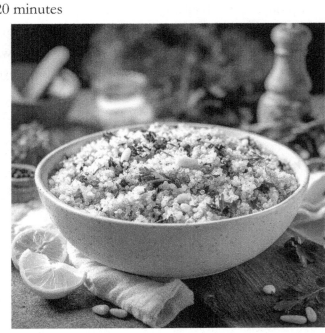

- 1 pound (450g) Brussels sprouts, trimmed and halved
- 2 tablespoons (30ml) olive oil
- 1/2 teaspoon (3g) salt
- 1/4 teaspoon (0.5g) black pepper
- 1/4 cup (60ml) balsamic vinegar
- 1 tablespoon (15ml) honey or maple syrup
- 2 tablespoons (20g) pine nuts (optional)

**INSTRUCTIONS:**

1. Set oven to 400°F (200°C).
2. Brussels sprouts should be combined with salt, pepper, and olive oil in a big bowl.
3. Spread Brussels sprouts on a baking sheet in a single layer, cut-side down. Roast, tossing occasionally, for 20 to 25 minutes or until the outside is crispy and the inside is soft.
4. Mix honey and balsamic vinegar in a small saucepan while the Brussels sprouts are roasting. Over medium heat, bring to a simmer and boil until slightly thickened, about 5 minutes.
5. After toasting pine nuts for two to three minutes over medium heat in a dry skillet, they should turn golden brown. Watch carefully to prevent burning.
6. Transfer roasted Brussels sprouts to a serving dish. Drizzle with balsamic glaze, then top with toasted pine nuts.

**Nutrition Per Serving:** Calories: 140 | Total Fat: 8g | Saturated Fat: 1g | Cholesterol: 0mg | Sodium: 320mg
Total Carbohydrate: 16g | Dietary Fiber: 4g | Sugars: 8g | Protein: 4g

## 90. Quinoa Pilaf with Herbs and Lemon

**Yields**: 4 servings | **Prep Time**: 10 minutes | **Cook Time**: 20 minutes

**Ingredients:**

- 1 cup (185g) quinoa, rinsed
- 2 cups (480ml) low-sodium vegetable broth
- 1 tablespoon (15ml) olive oil
- 1 small onion, finely chopped
- 2 cloves garlic, minced
- 1/4 cup (15g) fresh parsley, chopped
- 2 tablespoons (8g) fresh mint, chopped
- 2 tablespoons (8g) fresh dill, chopped
- Zest of 1 lemon
- 2 tablespoons (30ml) lemon juice
- 1/4 cup (35g) toasted pine nuts or sliced almonds
- 1/4 teaspoon (1.5g) salt
- 1/4 teaspoon (0.5g) black pepper

## INSTRUCTIONS:

1. Combine quinoa and vegetable broth in a medium saucepan. After bringing to a boil, lower heat, cover, and simmer the quinoa for 15 - 20 minutes, or until the liquid is absorbed and the quinoa is fluffy.
2. In a small skillet over medium heat, warm the olive oil while the quinoa cooks. Simmer the onion and garlic for 5 minutes or until soft.
3. In a large bowl, fluff the cooked quinoa with a fork. Add sautéed onion and garlic, chopped herbs, lemon zest, lemon juice, toasted nuts, salt, and pepper.
4. Gently toss all ingredients together until well combined.
5. Enjoy warm or at room temperature.

**Nutrition Per Serving:** Calories: 220 | Total Fat: 10g | Saturated Fat: 1g | Cholesterol: 0mg | Sodium: 220mg
Total Carbohydrate: 28g | Dietary Fiber: 4g | Sugars: 2g | Protein: 7g

## 91. Steamed Green Beans with Almonds

**Yields**: 4 servings | **Prep Time**: 10 minutes | **Cook Time**: 5-7 minutes

### Ingredients:

- 1 pound (450g) fresh green beans, trimmed
- 2 tablespoons (30ml) extra virgin olive oil
- 1/4 cup (35g) sliced almonds
- 1 clove garlic, minced
- 1 tablespoon (15ml) lemon juice
- 1/4 teaspoon (1.5g) salt
- 1/4 teaspoon (0.5g) black pepper
- Optional: 2 tablespoons (8g) fresh parsley, chopped

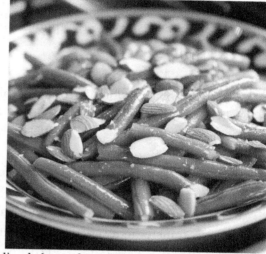

### INSTRUCTIONS:

1. Place green beans in a steamer basket over boiling water. Once crisp-tender, cover and steam for 5-7 minutes.
2. Heat a small skillet over medium heat while beans are steaming. Add sliced almonds and toast, stirring frequently, until golden brown, about 3-4 minutes. Remove from heat and set aside.
3. In a small bowl, whisk together olive oil, minced garlic, lemon juice, salt, and pepper.
4. Transfer green beans to a serving bowl once they are done. After adding the dressing, carefully mix the warm beans to coat. Sprinkle toasted almonds over the green beans. If using, add chopped parsley.

**Nutrition Per Serving:** Calories: 140 | Total Fat: 11g | Saturated Fat: 1.5g | Cholesterol: 0mg | Sodium: 150mg
Total Carbohydrate: 10g | Dietary Fiber: 4g | Sugars: 4g | Protein: 4g

# 92. Roasted Root Vegetables

**Yields**: 6 servings | **Prep Time**: 15 minutes | **Cook Time**: 40-45 minutes

**Ingredients:**

- 2 medium carrots, peeled and cut into 1-inch pieces
- 2 medium parsnips, peeled and cut into 1-inch pieces
- 1 large sweet potato, peeled and cut into 1-inch cubes
- 1 medium red onion, cut into wedges
- 1 medium beetroot, peeled and cut into 1-inch cubes
- 3 tablespoons (45ml) olive oil
- 2 cloves garlic, minced
- 1 tablespoon (6g) fresh rosemary, chopped
- 1 tablespoon (6g) fresh thyme leaves
- 1 teaspoon (6g) salt
- 1/2 teaspoon (1g) black pepper
- 2 tablespoons (30ml) balsamic vinegar
- Optional: 2 tablespoons (16g) pumpkin seeds for garnish

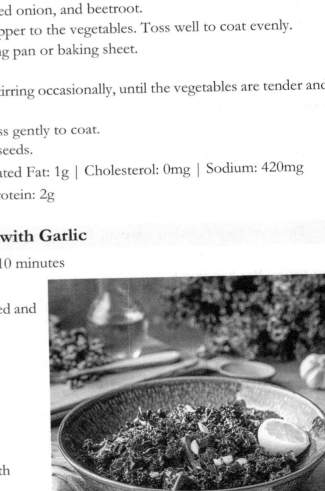

## INSTRUCTIONS:

1. Set oven to 425°F (220°C).
2. In a large bowl, combine carrots, parsnips, sweet potato, red onion, and beetroot.
3. Add olive oil, minced garlic, rosemary, thyme, salt, and pepper to the vegetables. Toss well to coat evenly.
4. Arrange the vegetables in a single layer on a sizable roasting pan or baking sheet.
5. Ensure they're not overcrowded.
6. Place in the preheated oven and roast for 40-45 minutes, stirring occasionally, until the vegetables are tender and have caramelized edges.
7. Remove from oven and drizzle with balsamic vinegar. Toss gently to coat.
8. If using, transfer to a serving dish and top with pumpkin seeds.

**Nutrition Per Serving:** Calories: 160 | Total Fat: 8g | Saturated Fat: 1g | Cholesterol: 0mg | Sodium: 420mg
Total Carbohydrate: 22g | Dietary Fiber: 5g | Sugars: 8g | Protein: 2g

# 93. Sautéed Kale with Garlic

**Yields**: 4 servings | **Prep Time**: 10 minutes | **Cook Time**: 10 minutes

**Ingredients:**

- 1 large bunch of kale (about 1 pound/450g), stems removed and leaves chopped
- 2 tablespoons (30ml) olive oil
- 3 cloves garlic, thinly sliced
- 1/4 teaspoon (1.5g) salt
- 1/4 teaspoon (0.5g) black pepper
- Pinch of red pepper flakes (optional)
- 1 tablespoon (15ml) lemon juice
- 2 tablespoons (30ml) water or low-sodium vegetable broth

## INSTRUCTIONS:

1. Wash kale leaves thoroughly. Slice the leaves into small pieces after removing the tough stems.
2. Olive oil should be heated to a medium temperature in a big skillet or wok.
3. When the oil is hot, add the sliced garlic and sauté it for approximately a minute, until it is fragrant but not browned.
4. Add chopped kale to the skillet. Add salt, pepper, and, if desired, red pepper flakes for seasoning. Stir to coat with oil and garlic.
5. Pour in water or vegetable broth. With the lid on, let the kale steam for around five minutes, stirring now and then.
6. Remove the lid and continue cooking, stirring frequently, until the kale is tender and the liquid has evaporated, about 2-3 more minutes. Remove from heat and stir in lemon juice.

**Nutrition Per Serving:** Calories: 100 | Total Fat: 7g | Saturated Fat: 1g | Cholesterol: 0mg | Sodium: 200mg
Total Carbohydrate: 8g | Dietary Fiber: 3g | Sugars: 2g | Protein: 3g

## 94. Brown Rice Pilaf with Mushrooms

**Yields**: 6 servings | **Prep Time**: 15 minutes | **Cook Time**: 45-50 minutes

### Ingredients:

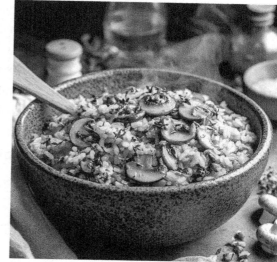

- 1 1/2 cups (300g) brown rice, rinsed
- 3 cups (720ml) low-sodium vegetable or chicken broth
- 2 tablespoons (30ml) olive oil
- 1 medium onion, finely chopped
- 2 cloves garlic, minced
- 8 ounces (225g) mushrooms (cremini or button), sliced
- 1 teaspoon (2g) dried thyme
- 1/2 teaspoon (3g) salt
- 1/4 teaspoon (0.5g) black pepper
- 1/4 cup (15g) fresh parsley, chopped
- 1/4 cup (30g) toasted sliced almonds (optional)

## INSTRUCTIONS:

1. Brown rice and broth should be combined in a medium saucepan. After bringing to a boil, lower the heat to a simmer, cover, and cook the rice for 40 to 45 minutes, or until it is soft and the liquid has been absorbed.
2. In a big skillet over medium heat, warm up the olive oil while the rice cooks. Simmer the onion and garlic for 5 minutes or until they are soft.
3. Add sliced mushrooms to the skillet. Cook for 8-10 minutes until mushrooms release their liquid and begin to brown.
4. Stir in dried thyme, salt, and pepper. Cook for another minute.
5. Once rice is cooked, fluff it with a fork and transfer to a large bowl. Add the mushroom mixture and chopped parsley. Stir gently to combine. If using, fold in toasted almonds.

**Nutrition Per Serving:** Calories: 220 | Total Fat: 7g | Saturated Fat: 1g | Cholesterol: 0mg | Sodium: 260mg
Total Carbohydrate: 35g | Dietary Fiber: 3g | Sugars: 2g | Protein: 5g

## 95. Roasted Carrots with Thyme

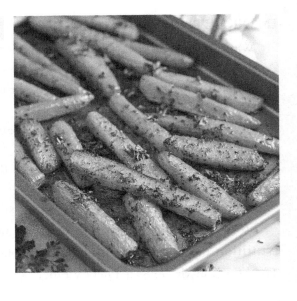

**Yields:** 4 servings | **Prep Time:** 10 minutes
**Cook Time:** 25-30 minutes

**Ingredients:**

- 1 pound (450g) medium carrots, peeled
- 2 tablespoons (30ml) olive oil
- 1 tablespoon (6g) fresh thyme leaves (or 1 teaspoon dried thyme)
- 1/2 teaspoon (3g) salt
- 1/4 teaspoon (0.5g) black pepper
- 1 tablespoon (15ml) honey (optional)
- 2 tablespoons (8g) fresh parsley, chopped (for garnish)

**INSTRUCTIONS:**

1. Set oven to 400°F (200°C).
2. If carrots are thick, halve them lengthwise; if not, leave whole.
   Cut into 2-inch pieces.
3. In a large bowl, toss carrots with olive oil, thyme, salt, and pepper until evenly coated.
4. Spread seasoned carrots in a single layer on a baking sheet.
5. Place in a preheated oven and roast for 20-25 minutes, stirring halfway through, until carrots are tender and lightly caramelized.
6. If using honey, drizzle it over the carrots and return to the oven for an additional 5 minutes.

**Nutrition Per Serving:** Calories: 110 | Total Fat: 7g | Saturated Fat: 1g | Cholesterol: 0mg | Sodium: 320mg

Total Carbohydrate: 12g | Dietary Fiber: 3g | Sugars: 6g | Protein: 1g

## 96. Baked Zucchini Chips

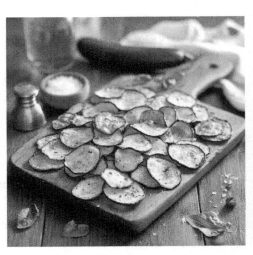

**Yields:** 4 servings | **Prep Time:** 15 minutes | **Cook Time:** 2-2.5 hours

**Ingredients:**

- 2 medium zucchini (about 1 pound/450g)
- 2 tablespoons (30ml) olive oil
- 1/2 teaspoon (3g) salt
- 1/4 teaspoon (0.5g) black pepper
- Optional: 1/4 teaspoon garlic powder or 1/2 teaspoon Italian seasoning

**INSTRUCTIONS:**

1. Set oven to 225°F (110°C). This low temperature helps dehydrate the zucchini without burning.
2. Wash and dry zucchini. Using a mandoline or sharp knife, slice zucchini into very thin rounds, about 1/8 inch thick.
3. Lay zucchini slices on paper towels and sprinkle with salt. After letting it sit for 10 minutes, pat dry to remove extra moisture.
4. In a large bowl, toss zucchini slices with olive oil, pepper, and any additional seasonings.
5. Place the zucchini slices on parchment paper-lined baking sheets in a single layer. Make sure slices don't overlap.
6. Place in preheated oven and bake for 2 to 2.5 hours, rotating pans halfway through. Chips are done when they're browned and crisp.
7. Remove from oven and let cool on the baking sheets for about 10 minutes to crisp up further.

**Nutrition Per Serving:** Calories: 70 | Total Fat: 7g | Saturated Fat: 1g | Cholesterol: 0mg | Sodium: 300mg
Total Carbohydrate: 3g | Dietary Fiber: 1g | Sugars: 2g | Protein: 1g

# 97. Braised Red Cabbage

**Yields:** 6 servings | **Prep Time:** 15 minutes | **Cook Time:** 45-50 minutes

**Ingredients:**

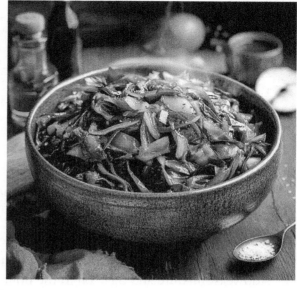

- 1 medium head red cabbage (about 2 pounds/900g), cored and thinly sliced
- 1 large onion, thinly sliced
- 2 medium apples, peeled, cored, and diced
- 2 tablespoons (30ml) olive oil
- 1/4 cup (60ml) apple cider vinegar
- 2 tablespoons (30ml) honey or maple syrup
- 1/2 cup (120ml) vegetable broth
- 1 teaspoon (2g) caraway seeds (optional)
- 1 bay leaf
- 1/2 teaspoon (3g) salt
- 1/4 teaspoon (0.5g) black pepper

## INSTRUCTIONS:

1. Thinly slice the cabbage and onion. Peel, core, and dice the apples.
2. In a large, heavy-bottomed pot or Dutch oven, heat olive oil over medium heat.
3. Add sliced onions and cook until softened, about 5 minutes.
4. Stir in the sliced cabbage and diced apples.
5. Pour in apple cider vinegar, honey (or maple syrup), and vegetable broth. Add caraway seeds (if using), bay leaf, salt, and pepper. Stir to combine.
6. Bring the mixture to a simmer, then reduce heat to low. Cook the cabbage, covered, stirring periodically, for 45 to 50 minutes or until it is soft.
7. Remove bay leaf. Taste and adjust seasoning if necessary.

**Nutrition Per Serving:** Calories: 120 | Total Fat: 5g | Saturated Fat: 1g | Cholesterol: 0mg | Sodium: 220mg
Total Carbohydrate: 20g | Dietary Fiber: 4g | Sugars: 14g | Protein: 2g

## 98. Whole Grain Dinner Rolls

**Yields:** 12 rolls | **Prep Time:** 20 minutes (plus 1 hour rising time) | **Cook Time:** 20-25 minutes

**Ingredients:**

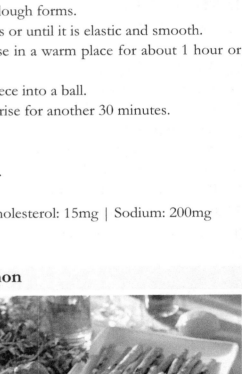

- 2 cups (240g) whole wheat flour
- 1 cup (120g) all-purpose flour
- 2 1/4 teaspoons (7g) active dry yeast
- 1 cup (240ml) warm water (110°F/43°C)
- 2 tablespoons (30ml) honey
- 2 tablespoons (30ml) olive oil
- 1 teaspoon (6g) salt
- 1 large egg, beaten (for egg wash)
- Optional: 1 tablespoon mixed seeds (sesame, poppy, flax) for topping

**INSTRUCTIONS:**

1. In a small bowl, combine warm water, honey, and yeast. Let sit for 5-10 minutes until frothy.
2. Mix the whole wheat flour, all-purpose flour, and salt in a sizable bowl.
3. Add yeast mixture and olive oil to the flour mixture. Stir until a shaggy dough forms.
4. After transferring the dough to a floured surface, knead it for 10 minutes or until it is elastic and smooth.
5. Place dough in a lightly oiled bowl, cover with a damp cloth, and let rise in a warm place for about 1 hour or until doubled in size.
6. Punch down the dough and divide it into 12 equal pieces. Shape each piece into a ball.
7. Place rolls on a baking sheet lined with parchment paper. Cover and let rise for another 30 minutes.
8. Set oven to 375°F (190°C).
9. Brush rolls with beaten egg and sprinkle with mixed seeds if using.
10. Place in preheated oven and bake for 20-25 minutes until golden brown.
11. Let rolls cool on a wire rack for at least 10 minutes before serving.

**Nutrition Per Roll:** Calories: 140 | Total Fat: 3g | Saturated Fat: 0.5g | Cholesterol: 15mg | Sodium: 200mg
Total Carbohydrate: 25g | Dietary Fiber: 3g | Sugars: 3g | Protein: 4g

## 99. Grilled Asparagus with Lemon

**Yields:** 4 servings | **Prep Time:** 5 minutes | **Cook Time:** 6-8 minutes

**Ingredients:**

- 1 pound (450g) fresh asparagus spears, trimmed
- 2 tablespoons (30ml) olive oil
- 1/2 teaspoon (3g) salt
- 1/4 teaspoon (0.5g) black pepper
- 1 lemon, halved
- Optional: 2 tablespoons (10g) grated Parmesan cheese

**INSTRUCTIONS:**

1. Preheat the grill to medium-high heat.
2. Wash asparagus and trim off the woody ends (about 1-2 inches from the bottom).
3. In a large shallow dish or on a baking sheet, toss asparagus with olive oil, salt, and pepper, ensuring all spears are evenly coated.
4. Place asparagus spears perpendicular to the grill grates. Grill for 6-8 minutes, turning occasionally, until tender-crisp and lightly charred.

5. Place lemon halves cut-side down on the grill for the last 2-3 minutes of cooking.
6. Remove asparagus and lemon from the grill. Squeeze grilled lemon over the asparagus.
7. Transfer to a serving platter. If using, sprinkle with grated Parmesan cheese.

**Nutrition Per Serving:** Calories: 80 | Total Fat: 7g | Saturated Fat: 1g | Cholesterol: 0mg | Sodium: 300mg
Total Carbohydrate: 5g | Dietary Fiber: 2g | Sugars: 2g | Protein: 3g

## 100. Roasted Beet and Carrot Medley

**Yields:** 4 servings | **Prep Time:** 15 minutes | **Cook Time:** 35-40 minutes

**Ingredients:**

- 3 medium beets (about 3/4 pound/340g), peeled and cut into 1-inch cubes
- 3 medium carrots (about 1/2 pound/225g), peeled and cut into 1-inch pieces
- 2 tablespoons (30ml) olive oil
- 1 tablespoon (15ml) balsamic vinegar
- 1 teaspoon (2g) fresh thyme leaves (or 1/2 teaspoon dried thyme)
- 1/2 teaspoon (3g) salt
- 1/4 teaspoon (0.5g) black pepper
- 2 tablespoons (16g) pumpkin seeds or chopped walnuts (optional)
- 2 tablespoons (8g) fresh parsley, chopped (for garnish)

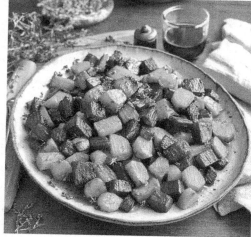

## INSTRUCTIONS:

1. Set oven to 400°F (200°C).
2. Peel and cut beets and carrots into roughly 1-inch pieces.
3. In a large bowl, toss beets and carrots with olive oil, balsamic vinegar, thyme, salt, and pepper.
4. Arrange the vegetables in a single layer on a parchment paper-lined baking sheet.
5. Place in a preheated oven and roast for 35-40 minutes, stirring halfway through, until vegetables are tender and slightly caramelized.
6. In a dry skillet over medium heat, toast walnuts or pumpkin seeds, if using, for two to three minutes or until aromatic.
7. Remove vegetables from oven, transfer to a serving dish, and sprinkle with toasted seeds and chopped parsley.

**Nutrition Per Serving:** Calories: 120 | Total Fat: 8g | Saturated Fat: 1g | Cholesterol: 0mg | Sodium: 340mg
Total Carbohydrate: 12g | Dietary Fiber: 3g | Sugars: 7g | Protein: 2g

# 101. Whole Wheat Couscous with Dried Fruit and Nuts

**Yields:** 6 servings | **Prep Time:** 10 minutes | **Cook Time:** 10 minutes

**Ingredients:**

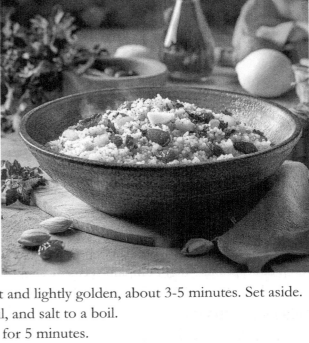

- 1 1/2 cups (270g) whole wheat couscous
- 1 3/4 cups (420ml) low-sodium vegetable or chicken broth
- 2 tablespoons (30ml) olive oil
- 1/2 teaspoon (3g) salt
- 1/4 cup (40g) dried apricots, chopped
- 1/4 cup (40g) dried cranberries or raisins
- 1/4 cup (30g) sliced almonds or chopped pistachios
- 2 tablespoons (8g) fresh mint, chopped
- 2 tablespoons (8g) fresh parsley, chopped
- Zest of 1 lemon
- 1 tablespoon (15ml) lemon juice
- 1/4 teaspoon (0.5g) ground cinnamon
- 1/4 teaspoon (0.5g) ground cumin

**INSTRUCTIONS:**

1. In a dry skillet over medium heat, toast the nuts until fragrant and lightly golden, about 3-5 minutes. Set aside.
2. In a medium saucepan, bring the broth, 1 tablespoon olive oil, and salt to a boil.
3. Remove pan from heat, stir in couscous, cover, and let stand for 5 minutes.
4. After 5 minutes, fluff the couscous with a fork.
5. Stir in dried fruit, toasted nuts, mint, parsley, lemon zest, lemon juice, cinnamon, and cumin.
6. After adding the final tablespoon of olive oil, gently toss to mix.

**Nutrition Per Serving:** Calories: 230 | Total Fat: 8g | Saturated Fat: 1g | Cholesterol: 0mg | Sodium: 220mg
Total Carbohydrate: 36g | Dietary Fiber: 5g | Sugars: 6g | Protein: 6g

---

## 5. Sweet Treats & Healthy Desserts
## 102. Baked Apples with Cinnamon and Oats

**Yields:** 4 servings | **Prep Time:** 15 minutes | **Cook Time:** 30-35 minutes

**Ingredients:**

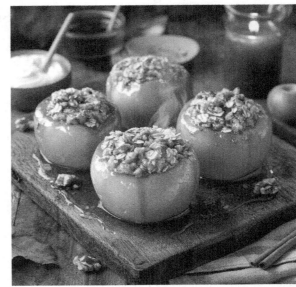

- 4 large baking apples (such as Honeycrisp, Granny Smith, or Braeburn)
- 1/4 cup (50g) rolled oats
- 2 tablespoons (25g) brown sugar
- 2 tablespoons (16g) chopped walnuts or pecans
- 1 teaspoon (2g) ground cinnamon
- 1/4 teaspoon (0.5g) ground nutmeg
- 2 tablespoons (30g) unsalted butter, softened
- 1/4 cup (60ml) apple juice or water
- Optional: Greek yogurt or vanilla ice cream for serving

**INSTRUCTIONS:**

1. Set oven to 375°F (190°C).
2. Wash apples and remove cores, leaving the bottom intact.
   Use a paring knife or apple corer, ensuring you don't cut through the bottom of the apple.

3. In a small bowl, mix oats, brown sugar, chopped nuts, cinnamon, nutmeg, and softened butter until well combined.

4. Spoon the oat mixture into the cored apples, pressing down gently.

5. Place stuffed apples in a baking dish. Fill the dish's bottom with water or apple juice.

6. Cover the dish with foil and bake for 20 minutes. After removing the foil, bake the apples for 10 to 15 minutes or until a fork easily pierces an apple.

7. Let cool for a few minutes before serving. Garnish with a tiny scoop of vanilla ice cream or a dollop of Greek yogurt, if you'd like.

**Nutrition Per Serving (without toppings):** Calories: 220 | Total Fat: 10g | Saturated Fat: 4g | Cholesterol: 15mg Sodium: 5mg | Total Carbohydrate: 34g | Dietary Fiber: 5g | Sugars: 24g | Protein: 2g

## 103. Greek Yogurt Panna Cotta with Berry Compote

**Yields**: 4 servings | **Prep Time**: 15 minutes | **Cook Time**: 5 minutes (plus 4 hours chilling time)

**Ingredients:**

**For the Panna Cotta:**

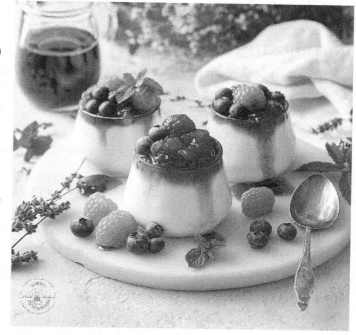

- 1 1/2 cups (360ml) plain Greek yogurt (2% or full-fat)
- 1 cup (240ml) low-fat milk
- 1/4 cup (60ml) honey
- 2 teaspoons (10ml) vanilla extract
- 2 1/4 teaspoons (7g) unflavored gelatin powder
- 3 tablespoons (45ml) cold water

**For the Berry Compote:**

- 2 cups (300g) mixed berries (strawberries, raspberries, blueberries)
- 2 tablespoons (30ml) honey
- 1 tablespoon (15ml) lemon juice
- 1/2 teaspoon (2g) cornstarch (optional, for thickening)

## INSTRUCTIONS:

**For the Panna Cotta:**

1. Sprinkle the gelatin over the cold water in a small bowl and allow it to bloom for 5 minutes.
2. In a saucepan, gently heat milk, honey, and vanilla until steaming (do not boil).
3. Take the milk mixture from the stove and whisk in the bloomed gelatin until it dissolves completely.
4. In a large bowl, whisk the Greek yogurt until smooth. Gradually whisk in the warm milk mixture until well combined.
5. Pour mixture into four ramekins or glasses. Refrigerate for at least 4 hours or overnight, covered with plastic wrap.

**For the Berry Compote:**

1. In a small saucepan, combine berries, honey, and lemon juice. Stirring occasionally, cook for approximately 5 minutes over medium heat.
2. If desired, mix cornstarch with 1 tablespoon water and stir into the berry mixture. Cook for an additional minute until slightly thickened.

**Nutrition Per Serving:** Calories: 250 | Total Fat: 6g | Saturated Fat: 4g | Cholesterol: 20mg | Sodium: 65mg Total Carbohydrate: 38g | Dietary Fiber: 2g | Sugars: 34g | Protein: 12g

## 104. Whole Grain Oatmeal Raisin Cookies

**Yields**: 24 cookies | **Prep Time**: 15 minutes | **Cook Time**: 12-15 minutes

**Ingredients:**

- 1 cup (120g) whole wheat flour
- 1 1/2 cups (135g) old-fashioned rolled oats
- 1/2 teaspoon (3g) baking soda
- 1 teaspoon (2g) ground cinnamon
- 1/4 teaspoon (1.5g) salt
- 1/2 cup (115g) unsalted butter, softened
- 1/2 cup (100g) brown sugar
- 1/4 cup (60ml) honey
- 1 large egg
- 1 teaspoon (5ml) vanilla extract
- 3/4 cup (120g) raisins
- Optional: 1/4 cup (30g) chopped walnuts

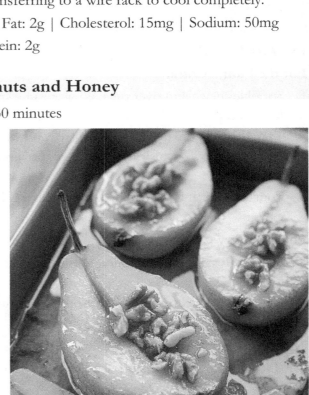

### INSTRUCTIONS:

1. Adjust the oven temperature to 350°F (175°C) and place parchment paper on two baking sheets.
2. Mix the oats, baking soda, cinnamon, and salt with the whole wheat flour in a medium-sized bowl.
3. Creamy butter, brown sugar, and honey should be combined in a big basin. Beat in the vanilla and egg until thoroughly blended.
4. Gradually stir the dry ingredients into the wet ingredients until just combined. Fold in raisins and walnuts (if using).
5. Round tablespoons of dough should be dropped, separated by around 2 inches, onto baking sheets that have been prepared.
6. Bake for 12 to 15 minutes in a preheated oven or until the edges are just beginning to turn brown.
7. Let cookies cool on the baking sheet for 5 minutes before transferring to a wire rack to cool completely.

**Nutrition Per Cookie:** Calories: 110 | Total Fat: 4g | Saturated Fat: 2g | Cholesterol: 15mg | Sodium: 50mg

Total Carbohydrate: 18g | Dietary Fiber: 2g | Sugars: 10g | Protein: 2g

## 105. Baked Pears with Walnuts and Honey

**Yields**: 4 servings | **Prep Time**: 10 minutes | **Cook Time**: 25-30 minutes

**Ingredients:**

- 4 ripe but firm pears (such as Bosc or Anjou)
- 1/4 cup (30g) chopped walnuts
- 2 tablespoons (30ml) honey, plus extra for drizzling
- 1 teaspoon (2g) ground cinnamon
- 1/4 teaspoon (0.5g) ground nutmeg
- 2 tablespoons (30g) unsalted butter, melted
- 1/4 cup (60ml) water
- Optional: Greek yogurt or vanilla ice cream for serving

## INSTRUCTIONS:

1. Set oven to 375°F (190°C).
2. Cut the pears in half lengthwise and remove the cores with a melon baller or tiny spoon.
3. Place pear halves cut side up in a baking dish.
4. In a small bowl, mix chopped walnuts, honey, cinnamon, and nutmeg.
5. Spoon the walnut mixture into the hollowed centers of each pear half.
6. Drizzle melted butter over the pears, then pour water into the bottom of the baking dish.
7. The pears should be soft when poked with a fork after 25 to 30 minutes of baking in a preheated oven.
8. Remove from oven and let cool for a few minutes. Drizzle with additional honey if desired.
9. Enjoy warm, optionally topped with a dollop of Greek yogurt or a small scoop of vanilla ice cream.

**Nutrition Per Serving (without optional toppings):** Calories: 220 | Total Fat: 11g | Saturated Fat: 4g Cholesterol: 15mg | Sodium: 5mg | Total Carbohydrate: 32g | Dietary Fiber: 5g | Sugars: 24g | Protein: 2g

## 106. Dark Chocolate Avocado Mousse

**Yields**: 4 servings | **Prep Time**: 15 minutes | **Chill Time**: At least 1 hour

### Ingredients:

- 2 ripe medium avocados, pitted and peeled
- 1/4 cup (60ml) unsweetened cocoa powder
- 1/4 cup (60ml) maple syrup or honey
- 1/4 cup (60ml) unsweetened almond milk (or any plant-based milk)
- 2 teaspoons (10ml) vanilla extract
- Pinch of salt
- Optional: 2 tablespoons (30ml) strong brewed coffee, cooled
- For garnish: Fresh berries, mint leaves, or a sprinkle of cocoa powder

### INSTRUCTIONS:

1. In a food processor or high-powered blender, combine avocados, cocoa powder, maple syrup, almond milk, vanilla extract, salt, and coffee (if using).
2. Blend until smooth, scraping down the sides as needed. It may take a few minutes to achieve a silky texture.
3. Taste the mousse and adjust sweetness if needed by adding more maple syrup.
4. Transfer the mousse to individual serving dishes or a large bowl. Cover the mousse with plastic wrap to prevent a skin from forming, pressing it firmly onto the surface.
   Allow it to set and chill in the refrigerator for at least 1 hour.
5. Before serving, garnish with fresh berries, mint leaves, or a light dusting of cocoa powder.

**Nutrition Per Serving:** Calories: 220 | Total Fat: 15g | Saturated Fat: 2g | Cholesterol: 0mg | Sodium: 40mg Total Carbohydrate: 22g | Dietary Fiber: 8g | Sugars: 11g | Protein: 3g

# 107. Whole Wheat Banana Bread

**Yields**: 1 loaf (12 slices) | **Prep Time**: 15 minutes | **Cook Time**: 50-60 minutes

**Ingredients:**

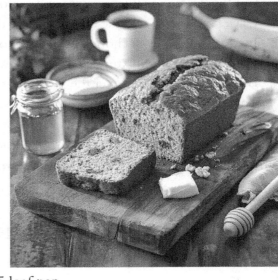

- 3 ripe bananas, mashed (about 1 1/2 cups)
- 1/3 cup (80ml) plain Greek yogurt
- 1/3 cup (80ml) honey or maple syrup
- 2 large eggs
- 1 teaspoon (5ml) vanilla extract
- 1 3/4 cups (210g) whole wheat flour
- 1 teaspoon (5g) baking soda
- 1/2 teaspoon (3g) salt
- 1 teaspoon (2g) ground cinnamon
- 1/4 cup (60ml) vegetable oil or melted coconut oil
- Optional: 1/2 cup (60g) chopped walnuts or pecans

**INSTRUCTIONS:**

1. Set oven to 350°F (175°C). Use parchment paper or grease a 9 x 5 loaf pan.
2. In a large bowl, mash the bananas. Add Greek yogurt, honey, eggs, and vanilla. Mix well.
3. Mix the baking soda, cinnamon, salt, and whole wheat flour in a separate basin.
4. Whisk the dry ingredients until they are just blended after adding them to the wet components. Fold in the oil and nuts (if using).
5. Pour batter into the prepared loaf pan. Bake for 50-60 minutes or until a toothpick inserted into the center comes out clean.
6. After 10 minutes of cooling in the pan, take out the bread and let it cool fully on a wire rack.

**Nutrition Per Slice:** Calories: 180 | Total Fat: 7g | Saturated Fat: 1g | Cholesterol: 30mg | Sodium: 180mg
Total Carbohydrate: 28g | Dietary Fiber: 3g | Sugars: 12g | Protein: 4g

# 108. Fruit Salad with Mint and Lime

**Yields**: 6 servings | **Prep Time**: 20 minutes | **Chill Time**: 30 minutes (optional)

**Ingredients:**

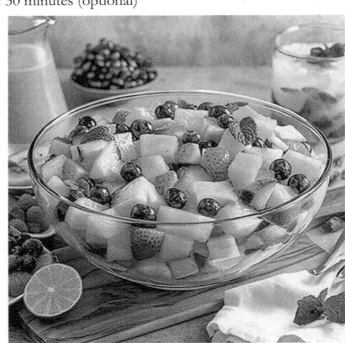

- 2 cups (300g) strawberries, hulled and quartered
- 2 cups (300g) fresh pineapple, cubed
- 2 cups (300g) cantaloupe or honeydew melon, cubed
- 1 cup (150g) blueberries
- 2 kiwis, peeled and sliced
- 1 large orange, peeled and segmented
- 2 tablespoons (30ml) fresh lime juice
- 2 tablespoons (30ml) honey
- 2 tablespoons (8g) fresh mint leaves, finely chopped
- Optional: 1/4 cup (30g) pomegranate seeds for garnish

## INSTRUCTIONS:

1. Wash and prepare all fruits as indicated, ensuring they are cut into bite-sized pieces.
2. Mix the lime juice and honey in a small bowl until thoroughly blended.
3. Gently toss all the prepared fruits together in a large bowl.
4. Pour the lime-honey dressing over the fruit and toss gently to coat.
5. Sprinkle chopped mint over the fruit salad and toss lightly to distribute.
6. If time allows, refrigerate for 30 minutes to let the flavors meld.
7. Before serving, give the salad a gentle toss. Garnish with pomegranate seeds if using.

**Nutrition Per Serving:** Calories: 120 | Total Fat: 0.5g | Saturated Fat: 0g | Cholesterol: 0mg | Sodium: 10mg
Total Carbohydrate: 30g | Dietary Fiber: 4g | Sugars: 24g | Protein: 1g

## 109. Almond Flour Blueberry Muffins

**Yields**: 12 muffins | **Prep Time**: 15 minutes | **Cook Time**: 20-25 minutes

**Ingredients:**

- 2 1/2 cups (240g) almond flour
- 1/4 cup (30g) coconut flour
- 1/2 teaspoon baking soda
- 1/4 teaspoon salt
- 3 large eggs
- 1/3 cup (80ml) honey or maple syrup
- 1/4 cup (60ml) unsweetened almond milk
- 1/4 cup (60ml) coconut oil, melted
- 1 teaspoon (5ml) vanilla extract
- 1 teaspoon (5ml) apple cider vinegar
- 1 cup (150g) fresh blueberries
- Optional: 1/2 teaspoon lemon zest

## INSTRUCTIONS:

1. Set oven to 350°F (175°C). Use paper liners or coconut oil to grease a 12-cup muffin pan.
2. In a large bowl, whisk together almond flour, coconut flour, baking soda, and salt.
3. In another bowl, whisk eggs, honey, almond milk, melted coconut oil, vanilla extract, and apple cider vinegar.
4. After adding the wet ingredients to the dry ingredients, thoroughly mix them.
5. Fold in blueberries and lemon zest (if using).
6. Evenly distribute the batter into the muffin tins, filling each to about 3/4 of the way.
7. Place in preheated oven and bake for 20-25 minutes, or until a toothpick inserted into the center comes out clean.
8. Let muffins cool in the tin for 5 minutes, then transfer to a wire rack to cool completely.

**Nutrition Per Muffin:** Calories: 220 | Total Fat: 17g | Saturated Fat: 5g | Cholesterol: 45mg | Sodium: 95mg
Total Carbohydrate: 14g | Dietary Fiber: 4g | Sugars: 8g | Protein: 7g

## 110. Poached Peaches with Yogurt

**Yields**: 4 servings | **Prep Time**: 10 minutes | **Cook Time**: 15-20 minutes

**Ingredients:**

**For the Poached Peaches:**

- 4 ripe but firm peaches, halved and pitted
- 2 cups (480ml) water
- 1/4 cup (50g) granulated sugar or honey
- 1 vanilla bean, split lengthwise (or 1 teaspoon vanilla extract)
- 1 cinnamon stick
- 2 strips of lemon zest

**For Serving:**

- 2 cups (480g) Greek yogurt
- 2 tablespoons (30ml) honey
- 1/4 cup (30g) chopped pistachios or sliced almonds (optional)
- Fresh mint leaves for garnish

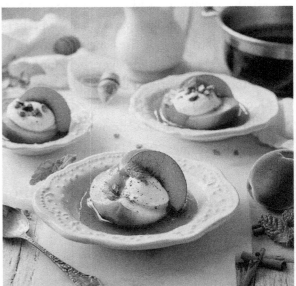

**INSTRUCTIONS:**

1. In a large saucepan, combine water, sugar, vanilla bean (or extract), cinnamon stick, and lemon zest. Over medium heat, bring to a simmer and whisk until sugar dissolves.
2. Gently place peach halves in the simmering liquid. Cook for 5-7 minutes for firm peaches or 3-5 minutes for softer peaches until they're tender when pierced with a knife.
3. Remove peaches with a slotted spoon and set aside to cool slightly. If desired, continue simmering the cooking liquid until reduced by half to create a syrup.
4. Mix Greek yogurt with honey in a small bowl until well combined.
5. Place two peach halves in each serving bowl. Top with a generous dollop of honeyed yogurt. Drizzle with reduced cooking syrup if using. Sprinkle with chopped nuts and garnish with fresh mint leaves.

**Nutrition Per Serving:** Calories: 220 | Total Fat: 6g | Saturated Fat: 3g | Cholesterol: 10mg | Sodium: 30mg

Total Carbohydrate: 35g | Dietary Fiber: 3g | Sugars: 31g | Protein: 11g

## 6. Snacks & Small Bites

## 111. Homemade Trail Mix

**Yields**: 2 servings (about 1/2 cup each) | **Prep Time**: 10 minutes

**Ingredients:**

- 1/4 cup (30g) raw almonds
- 1/4 cup (30g) raw walnuts
- 2 tablespoons (20g) pumpkin seeds
- 2 tablespoons (20g) sunflower seeds
- 2 tablespoons (20g) dried cranberries
- 2 tablespoons (20g) dried blueberries
- 2 tablespoons (10g) unsweetened coconut flakes
- 1 tablespoon (15g) dark chocolate chips (70% cocoa or higher)

**INSTRUCTIONS:**

1. Mix all ingredients in a medium bowl.
2. Transfer the mix to an airtight container or portion into individual servings in small zip-lock bags.

**Nutrition Per Serving:** Calories: 320 | Total Fat: 24g | Saturated Fat: 5g | Cholesterol: 0mg | Sodium: 5mg

Total Carbohydrate: 22g | Dietary Fiber: 6g | Sugars: 12g | Protein: 9g

## 112. Whole Grain Crackers with Hummus

**Yields**: 2 servings | **Prep Time**: 15 minutes (if making homemade hummus)

**Ingredients:**

**For the Hummus:**

- 1 can (15 oz/425g) chickpeas, drained and rinsed
- 2 tablespoons (30ml) tahini
- 2 tablespoons (30ml) extra virgin olive oil
- 2 tablespoons (30ml) lemon juice
- 1 small garlic clove, minced
- 1/4 teaspoon salt
- 2-3 tablespoons water (as needed for consistency)

**For Serving:**

- 1 cup (about 30g) whole grain crackers
- Optional: Cucumber slices, cherry tomatoes, or carrot sticks for dipping

**INSTRUCTIONS:**

1. In a food processor, combine chickpeas, tahini, olive oil, lemon juice, garlic, and salt. Process until smooth, adding water as needed to reach desired consistency.
2. Taste and adjust salt, lemon juice, or garlic as needed.
3. Divide hummus between two small bowls. Serve with whole-grain crackers and optional vegetable slices.

**Nutrition Per Serving (including 1/2 cup hummus and 1/2 cup crackers):**

Calories: 300 | Total Fat: 18g | Saturated Fat: 2g | Cholesterol: 0mg | Sodium: 400mg
Total Carbohydrate: 30g | Dietary Fiber: 8g | Sugars: 2g | Protein: 10g

## 113. Apple Slices with Almond Butter

**Yields**: 2 servings | **Prep Time**: 5 minutes

**Ingredients:**

- 2 medium apples (preferably a crisp variety like Honeycrisp or Granny Smith)
- 4 tablespoons (64g) natural almond butter
- Optional: 1 teaspoon cinnamon
- Optional: 1 tablespoon (10g) chia seeds or chopped nuts for topping

**INSTRUCTIONS:**

1. Wash and core the apples. Cut each apple into 8 slices.
2. Divide the apple slices between two plates.
3. Spread or dollop 2 tablespoons of almond butter onto the apple slices on each plate.
4. If desired, sprinkle cinnamon, chia seeds, or chopped nuts over the almond butter.

**Nutrition Per Serving:** Calories: 270 | Total Fat: 18g | Saturated Fat: 1.5g | Cholesterol: 0mg | Sodium: 3mg
Total Carbohydrate: 25g | Dietary Fiber: 7g | Sugars: 16g | Protein: 8g

# 114. Roasted Chickpeas

**Yields:** 2 servings | **Prep Time:** 5 minutes | **Cook Time:** 25-30 minutes

**Ingredients:**

- 1 can (15 oz/425g) chickpeas, drained and rinsed
- 1 tablespoon (15ml) olive oil
- 1/2 teaspoon salt
- 1 teaspoon spice mix of choice (options: cumin, paprika, garlic powder, curry powder, or za'atar)

## INSTRUCTIONS:

1. Set oven to 400°F (200°C).
2. Drain and rinse chickpeas. Pat them dry with a clean kitchen towel or paper towels, removing any loose skins.
3. In a bowl, toss chickpeas with olive oil, salt, and your chosen spice mix until evenly coated.
4. Spread chickpeas in a single layer on a baking sheet.
5. Place in the preheated oven and bake for 25 to 30 minutes, until the chickpeas are brown and crispy, shaking the pan halfway through.
6. Let cool for 5-10 minutes before serving. They will become crispier as they cool.

**Nutrition Per Serving:** Calories: 180 | Total Fat: 8g | Saturated Fat: 1g | Cholesterol: 0mg | Sodium: 600mg

Total Carbohydrate: 22g | Dietary Fiber: 6g | Sugars: 4g | Protein: 7g

# 115. Vegetable Sticks with Greek Yogurt Dip

**Yields**: 2 servings | **Prep Time:** 15 minutes

**Ingredients:**

**For the Vegetable Sticks:**

- 1 medium carrot, cut into sticks
- 1 medium cucumber, cut into sticks
- 1 red bell pepper, cut into strips
- 2 celery stalks, cut into sticks

**For the Greek Yogurt Dip:**

- 1 cup (245g) plain Greek yogurt
- 1 tablespoon (15ml) lemon juice
- 1 small garlic clove, minced
- 1 tablespoon fresh dill, finely chopped (or 1 teaspoon dried dill)
- 1/4 teaspoon salt
- 1/8 teaspoon black pepper

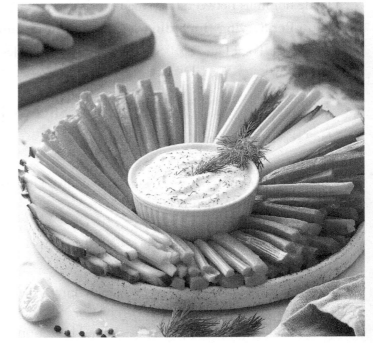

## INSTRUCTIONS:

1. Wash and cut all vegetables into sticks or strips of similar size.
2. In a small bowl, combine Greek yogurt, lemon juice, minced garlic, dill, salt, and pepper. Mix well.
3. Refrigerate the dip for at least 30 minutes to allow flavors to meld (if time permits).
4. Divide the vegetable sticks between two plates and serve with the yogurt dip.

**Nutrition Per Serving (including half of the dip):** Calories: 140 | Total Fat: 4g | Saturated Fat: 2.5g

Cholesterol: 15mg | Sodium: 350mg | Total Carbohydrate: 14g | Dietary Fiber: 3g | Sugars: 8g | Protein: 13g

# Part 3: Meal Planning and Prep

## 8-Week Meal Plan

**Introduction:**

This 8-week meal plan is designed to help you incorporate the recipes from this cookbook into your daily life, ensuring a balanced and diverticulosis-friendly diet. Each week includes a variety of meals that cater to different stages of diverticulosis management, from gentle options for sensitive days to fiber-rich choices for maintaining gut health.

Before making any significant dietary adjustments, remember to consult your healthcare practitioner and modify portion sizes to suit your individual needs. You are welcome to switch up the recipes or make your favorites again. Remember to check your pantry before shopping to avoid buying items you already have, and adjust quantities based on your household size and any dietary restrictions.

### Week 1: Gentle Nourishment

|  | Breakfast | Lunch | Dinner | Snack |
|---|---|---|---|---|
| **Monday** | Well-Cooked Rice Pudding (8) | Soothing Bone Broth with Ginger and Turmeric (1) | Simple Poached Salmon (13) | Gelatin with Pear Juice (6) |
| **Tuesday** | Soft-Boiled Eggs on White Toast (12) | Clear Chicken Broth with Soft Noodles (2) | Plain Poached Chicken Breast (14) | Steamed Zucchini Puree (7) |
| **Wednesday** | Well-Cooked White Rice (11) | Egg Drop Soup (3) | Tender Flaked White Fish (15) | Smooth Mashed Potatoes (Without Skin) (10) |
| **Thursday** | White Rice Congee with Chicken (9) | Tofu and Broth Soup (4) | Steamed White Fish with Lemon (16) | Well-Cooked Rice Pudding (8) |
| **Friday** | Soft-Boiled Eggs on White Toast (12) | Pureed Carrot Soup (5) | Simple Poached Salmon (13) | Gelatin with Pear Juice (6) |
| **Saturday** | Well-Cooked White Rice (11) | Soothing Bone Broth with Ginger and Turmeric (1) | Plain Poached Chicken Breast (14) | Steamed Zucchini Puree (7) |
| **Sunday** | White Rice Congee with Chicken (9) | Clear Chicken Broth with Soft Noodles (2) | Tender Flaked White Fish (15) | Smooth Mashed Potatoes (Without Skin) (10) |

### Week 2: Gradually Adding Back Fiber

|  | Breakfast | Lunch | Dinner | Snack |
|---|---|---|---|---|
| **Monday** | Scrambled Eggs with Spinach (17) | Chicken and Rice Soup with Carrots and Dill (19) | Baked Cod with Mashed Sweet Potatoes (23) | Applesauce Pancakes (20) |
| **Tuesday** | Easy-to-Digest Oatmeal with Banana and Cinnamon (26) | Creamy Butternut Squash Soup (Strained) (27) | Ground Turkey and Rice Bowl (28) | Mashed Cauliflower with Herbs (21) |
| **Wednesday** | Banana Oatmeal Smoothie (22) | Salmon Patties (No Breadcrumbs) (24) | Tofu and Vegetable Curry (Mild) (25) | Baked Sweet Potato (31) |
| **Thursday** | Scrambled Eggs with Canned Peaches (18) | Baked Chicken Breast with Mashed Carrots (29) | Well-Cooked Lentil Soup (Pureed) (33) | Poached Pears in Ginger Tea (30) |
| **Friday** | Creamy Coconut Chia Seed Pudding (32) | Chicken and Rice Soup with Carrots and Dill (19) | Baked Cod with Mashed Sweet Potatoes (23) | Applesauce Pancakes (20) |
| **Saturday** | Easy-to-Digest Oatmeal with Banana and Cinnamon (26) | Salmon Patties (No Breadcrumbs) (24) | Ground Turkey and Rice Bowl (28) | Baked Sweet Potato (31) |
| **Sunday** | Banana Oatmeal Smoothie (22) | Creamy Butternut Squash Soup (Strained) (27) | Tofu and Vegetable Curry (Mild) (25) | Creamy Coconut Chia Seed Pudding (32) |

## Week 3: Increasing Fiber and Variety

|  | Breakfast | Lunch | Dinner | Snack |
|---|---|---|---|---|
| **Monday** | High-Fiber Berry Blast Smoothie (34) | Lentil and Vegetable Soup (49) | Slow Cooker Chicken and Vegetable Stew (69) | Whole Grain Crackers with Hummus (112) |
| **Tuesday** | Overnight Oats with Berries and Nuts (35) | Greek Salad with Grilled Chicken (52) | Baked Salmon with Dill Sauce (77) | Apple Slices with Almond Butter (113) |
| **Wednesday** | Spinach and Feta Egg White Omelet (36) | Minestrone Soup with Whole Wheat Pasta (51) | Turkey Meatloaf with Oats (70) | Roasted Chickpeas (114) |
| **Thursday** | Apple Cinnamon Oatmeal with Flaxseed (38) | Roasted Chickpea and Quinoa Salad (50) | Shrimp and Vegetable Skewers (78) | Vegetable Sticks with Greek Yogurt Dip (115) |
| **Friday** | Avocado Toast on Whole Grain Bread (40) | Butternut Squash and Apple Soup (53) | Grilled Pork Tenderloin with Apple Chutney (71) | Homemade Trail Mix (111) |
| **Saturday** | Greek Yogurt Parfait with Berries and Granola (39) | Spinach and Strawberry Salad with Poppy Seed Dressing (54) | Beef and Broccoli Stir-Fry with Brown Rice (72) | Baked Apples with Cinnamon and Oats (102) |
| **Sunday** | Quinoa Breakfast Bowl with Fresh Fruit (42) | Turkey and Bean Chili (55) | Cod Fish Tacos with Cabbage Slaw (81) | Whole Grain Oatmeal Raisin Cookies (104) |

## Week 4: Embracing High-Fiber Lifestyle

|  | Breakfast | Lunch | Dinner | Snack |
|---|---|---|---|---|
| **Monday** | Whole Grain Pancakes with Berry Compote (43) | Kale and Roasted Vegetable Salad (56) | Lentil and Mushroom Loaf (83) | Dark Chocolate Avocado Mousse (106) |
| **Tuesday** | Tofu Scramble with Vegetables (48) | Carrot and Ginger Soup (57) | Grilled Trout with Lemon and Herbs (80) | Fruit Salad with Mint and Lime (108) |
| **Wednesday** | Buckwheat Porridge with Cinnamon and Pear (47) | Tabbouleh Salad with Quinoa (58) | Turkey and Spinach Stuffed Bell Peppers (74) | Almond Flour Blueberry Muffins (109) |
| **Thursday** | Breakfast Burrito with Whole Wheat Tortilla (45) | Split Pea Soup with Ham (59) | Chickpea and Spinach Curry (85) | Baked Pears with Walnuts and Honey (105) |
| **Friday** | Pumpkin Spice Smoothie Bowl (41) | Asian-Inspired Cabbage Salad (60) | Baked Tilapia with Tomato and Olive Topping (82) | Whole Wheat Banana Bread (107) |
| **Saturday** | Baked Oatmeal with Apples and Walnuts (44) | Grilled Vegetable and Chickpea Salad (62) | Greek Yogurt Panna Cotta with Berry Compote (103) | Greek Yogurt Panna Cotta with Berry Compote (103) |
| **Sunday** | Whole Grain English Muffin with Egg and Spinach (46) | Mediterranean Couscous Salad (66) | Black Bean and Sweet Potato Tacos (88) | Poached Peaches with Yogurt (110) |

# Week 5-8: Maintaining a High-Fiber Lifestyle

|  | Breakfast | Lunch | Dinner | Snack |
|---|---|---|---|---|
| **Monday** | Peach and Ginger Smoothie (37) | Tomato and Basil Soup with Whole Grain Croutons (61) | Baked Chicken Fajitas (73) | Roasted Chickpeas (114) |
| **Tuesday** | Avocado Toast on Whole Grain Bread (40) | Southwest Black Bean and Corn Salad (64) | Grilled Lemon Herb Chicken (75) | Apple Slices with Almond Butter (113) |
| **Wednesday** | Greek Yogurt Parfait with Berries and Granola (39) | Mushroom and Barley Soup (63) | Shrimp and Vegetable Skewers (78) | Whole Grain Crackers with Hummus (112) |
| **Thursday** | Spinach and Feta Egg White Omelet (36) | White Bean and Kale Soup (67) | Beef and Barley Casserole (76) | Baked Zucchini Chips (96) |
| **Friday** | Apple Cinnamon Oatmeal with Flaxseed (38) | Tuna Nicoise Salad (79) | Vegetable and Tofu Stir-Fry (87) | Fruit Salad with Mint and Lime (108) |
| **Saturday** | Whole Grain Pancakes with Berry Compote (43) | Zucchini and Leek Soup (65) | Baked Salmon with Dill Sauce (77) | Whole Grain Oatmeal Raisin Cookies (104) |
| **Sunday** | Tofu Scramble with Vegetables (48) | Beet and Goat Cheese Salad with Walnuts (68) | Turkey and Bean Chili (55) | Dark Chocolate Avocado Mousse (106) |

# Week 6

|  | Breakfast | Lunch | Dinner | Snack |
|---|---|---|---|---|
| **Monday** | Overnight Oats with Berries and Nuts (35) | Carrot and Ginger Soup (57) | Stuffed Portobello Mushrooms (84) | Vegetable Sticks with Greek Yogurt Dip (115) |
| **Tuesday** | Pumpkin Spice Smoothie Bowl (41) | Greek Salad with Grilled Chicken (52) | Black Bean and Sweet Potato Tacos (88) | Homemade Trail Mix (111) |
| **Wednesday** | Whole Grain English Muffin with Egg and Spinach (46) | Lentil and Vegetable Soup (49) | Grilled Trout with Lemon and Herbs (80) | Baked Apples with Cinnamon and Oats (102) |
| **Thursday** | High-Fiber Berry Blast Smoothie (34) | Mediterranean Couscous Salad (66) | Turkey Meatloaf with Oats (70) | Almond Flour Blueberry Muffins (109) |
| **Friday** | Buckwheat Porridge with Cinnamon and Pear (47) | Spinach and Strawberry Salad with Poppy Seed Dressing (54) | Cod Fish Tacos with Cabbage Slaw (81) | Poached Peaches with Yogurt (110) |
| **Saturday** | Quinoa Breakfast Bowl with Fresh Fruit (42) | Asian-Inspired Cabbage Salad (60) | Chickpea and Spinach Curry (85) | Whole Wheat Banana Bread (107) |
| **Sunday** | Baked Oatmeal with Apples and Walnuts (44) | Roasted Chickpea and Quinoa Salad (50) | Slow Cooker Chicken and Vegetable Stew (69) | Greek Yogurt Panna Cotta with Berry Compote (103) |

## Week 7

|  | Breakfast | Lunch | Dinner | Snack |
|---|---|---|---|---|
| **Monday** | Breakfast Burrito with Whole Wheat Tortilla (45) | Butternut Squash and Apple Soup (53) | Lentil and Mushroom Loaf (83) | Baked Pears with Walnuts and Honey (105) |
| **Tuesday** | Peach and Ginger Smoothie (37) | Kale and Roasted Vegetable Salad (56) | Baked Tilapia with Tomato and Olive Topping (82) | Roasted Chickpeas (114) |
| **Wednesday** | Avocado Toast on Whole Grain Bread (40) | Split Pea Soup with Ham (59) | Grilled Pork Tenderloin with Apple Chutney (71) | Apple Slices with Almond Butter (113) |
| **Thursday** | Greek Yogurt Parfait with Berries and Granola (39) | Tabbouleh Salad with Quinoa (58) | Quinoa-Stuffed Acorn Squash (86) | Whole Grain Crackers with Hummus (112) |
| **Friday** | Spinach and Feta Egg White Omelet (36) | Minestrone Soup with Whole Wheat Pasta (51) | Beef and Broccoli Stir-Fry with Brown Rice (72) | Fruit Salad with Mint and Lime (108) |
| **Saturday** | Apple Cinnamon Oatmeal with Flaxseed (38) | Grilled Vegetable and Chickpea Salad (62) | Turkey and Spinach Stuffed Bell Peppers (74) | Whole Grain Oatmeal Raisin Cookies (104) |
| **Sunday** | Tofu Scramble with Vegetables (48) | White Bean and Kale Soup (67) | Shrimp and Vegetable Skewers (78) | Dark Chocolate Avocado Mousse (106) |

## Week 8

|  | Breakfast | Lunch | Dinner | Snack |
|---|---|---|---|---|
| **Monday** | Overnight Oats with Berries and Nuts (35) | Zucchini and Leek Soup (65) | Baked Salmon with Dill Sauce (77) | Vegetable Sticks with Greek Yogurt Dip (115) |
| **Tuesday** | Pumpkin Spice Smoothie Bowl (41) | Southwest Black Bean and Corn Salad (64) | Vegetable and Tofu Stir-Fry (87) | Homemade Trail Mix (111) |
| **Wednesday** | Whole Grain English Muffin with Egg and Spinach (46) | Carrot and Ginger Soup (57) | Grilled Lemon Herb Chicken (75) | Baked Apples with Cinnamon and Oats (102) |
| **Thursday** | High-Fiber Berry Blast Smoothie (34) | Beet and Goat Cheese Salad with Walnuts (68) | Black Bean and Sweet Potato Tacos (88) | Almond Flour Blueberry Muffins (109) |
| **Friday** | Buckwheat Porridge with Cinnamon and Pear (47) | Tomato and Basil Soup with Whole Grain Croutons (61) | Cod Fish Tacos with Cabbage Slaw (81) | Poached Peaches with Yogurt (110) |
| **Saturday** | Quinoa Breakfast Bowl with Fresh Fruit (42) | Mediterranean Couscous Salad (66) | Turkey Meatloaf with Oats (70) | Whole Wheat Banana Bread (107) |
| **Sunday** | Baked Oatmeal with Apples and Walnuts (44) | Mushroom and Barley Soup (63) | Chickpea and Spinach Curry (85) | Greek Yogurt Panna Cotta with Berry Compote (103) |

## Tips for Using This Meal Plan:

1. Adjust portion sizes as needed to suit your individual requirements.
2. Feel free to swap recipes or repeat favorites based on your preferences and tolerances.
3. Always listen to your body and consult your healthcare provider if you have concerns.
4. Use leftovers creatively to minimize food waste and save time.
5. Prep ingredients in advance when possible to make weekday cooking easier.

Remember, this meal plan is a guide to help you implement the recipes from this cookbook into your daily life. It's designed to support your journey in managing diverticulosis through diet, providing structure while allowing for flexibility to suit your individual needs.

# Batch Cooking Guide: Cook Once, Eat All Week

To save time, batch cooking involves preparing larger quantities of food ingredients all at once. These components can then be combined and served in different combinations throughout the week to make a variety of wholesome meals. Those managing diverticulosis will find this strategy especially helpful, as it ensures that there are always options that are gentle on the stomach.

## Key Components to Batch Cook:

1. Whole Grains: Cook a large batch of brown rice, quinoa, or barley. These can be used as bases for bowls, added to soups, or served as sides.
2. Lean Proteins: Grill or bake several chicken breasts, prepare a large batch of turkey meatballs, or cook a pot of lentils. These can be added to salads, sandwiches, or main dishes.
3. Roasted Vegetables: Roast a range of veggies, including carrots, Brussels sprouts, and sweet potatoes.
4. These can be used in salads, side dishes, or grain bowls.
5. Soups and Stews: Make a big pot of stew or soup that you can split out and freeze for easy dinners.
6. Prepared Salads: Make sturdy salads like quinoa tabbouleh or bean salads that keep well in the refrigerator.

## Step-by-Step Batch Cooking Process:

1. Plan Your Menu: Choose 3-4 recipes from the cookbook that share common ingredients.
2. Prep Ingredients: Wash, chop, and prepare all vegetables and proteins.
3. Cook Grains: Start with grains, which often take the longest to cook.
4. Roast Vegetables: Roast a large tray of mixed vegetables while the grains are cooking.
5. Prepare Proteins: Grill, bake, or cook your chosen proteins.
6. Make a Soup or Stew: Utilize any remaining vegetables or proteins in a large batch of soup.
7. Prepare Sauces and Dressings: Make 2-3 different sauces or dressings to vary your meals throughout the week.
8. Cool and Store: Before putting any ingredients in sealed freezer or refrigerator containers, allow them all to cool completely.

## Sample Batch Cooking Plan:

1. Cook: Brown rice, quinoa, roasted mixed vegetables, grilled chicken breasts, lentil soup, and prepare a large Greek salad.
2. Potential Meals:

 - Monday: Quinoa bowl with roasted vegetables and grilled chicken
 - Tuesday: Lentil soup with a side of Greek salad
 - Wednesday: Brown rice stir-fry with leftover vegetables and chicken
 - Thursday: Greek salad topped with quinoa and lentils
 - Friday: Chicken and rice soup (using leftover chicken, rice, and vegetables)

Store your batch-cooked items properly and consume refrigerated items within 3-4 days. Frozen items can typically last up to 3 months.

You can ensure that you always have wholesome, diverticulosis-friendly foods on hand by incorporating batch cooking into your weekly routine. This will make it simpler to keep a balanced diet even on hectic days.

## Tips for Eating Out with Diverticulosis

Dining out can be enjoyable while managing diverticulosis with some careful planning. Always prioritize high-fiber, gut-friendly options when available. Choose restaurants that offer whole-grain bread, brown rice, or quinoa as alternatives to refined grains. Opt for grilled, baked, or steamed dishes instead of fried foods. Soups, especially those with vegetables or legumes, can be excellent choices. Ask for dressing on the side, and make sure your salad has a range of vibrant veggies. When planning main courses, opt for fish, skinless poultry, or plant-based proteins, and serve them with steamed vegetables or a baked potato with the skin. Be cautious with spicy foods if they trigger symptoms. Never hesitate to ask your server to adjust the meal to fit your dietary requirements or to substitute an ingredient. Remember to eat slowly, chew thoroughly, and stay well-hydrated. If you're unsure about a menu item, ask for more information or choose a simpler dish. Lastly, consider eating a small, fiber-rich snack before going out to avoid overindulging in less suitable options.

## CONCLUSION

Throughout this cookbook, we've journeyed from understanding diverticulosis to managing acute flare-ups, and finally to embracing a gut-healthy lifestyle. You've been equipped with a variety of delicious recipes, practical meal plans, and strategies for maintaining your diet even when eating out or pressed for time.

Remember, you have the power to significantly impact your gut health through the food choices you make every day. The recipes and plans in this book are not rigid rules but flexible guidelines that you can adapt to your personal tastes and needs. Listen to your body and work with your healthcare provider to find what works best for you.

Changing your diet is a process that requires patience and persistence. You may not see dramatic changes overnight, but with consistent effort, you're likely to experience improvements in your symptoms and overall well-being.

Living with diverticulosis doesn't mean a life of bland, restricted eating. As you've seen in these pages, a gut-friendly diet can be varied, flavorful, and satisfying. By incorporating these recipes and principles into your daily life, you're not just managing a condition – you're nourishing your body, expanding your culinary horizons, and taking proactive steps toward better health.

Here's to your journey towards a happier, healthier gut. Bon appétit!

Morgan Alexandra

**"Thank you for dedicating your time to exploring this book.** We genuinely value your thoughts, insights, and feedback. Your unique perspective not only aids fellow readers in determining if this book suits them but also offers invaluable guidance to the author. Every opinion holds significance, and we eagerly anticipate hearing yours."

amazon.com     amazon.co.uk     amazon.ca     mazon.com.au

# INDEX

# Your Notes and Recipe Modifications

Made in the USA
Monee, IL
25 October 2024

68656008R00063